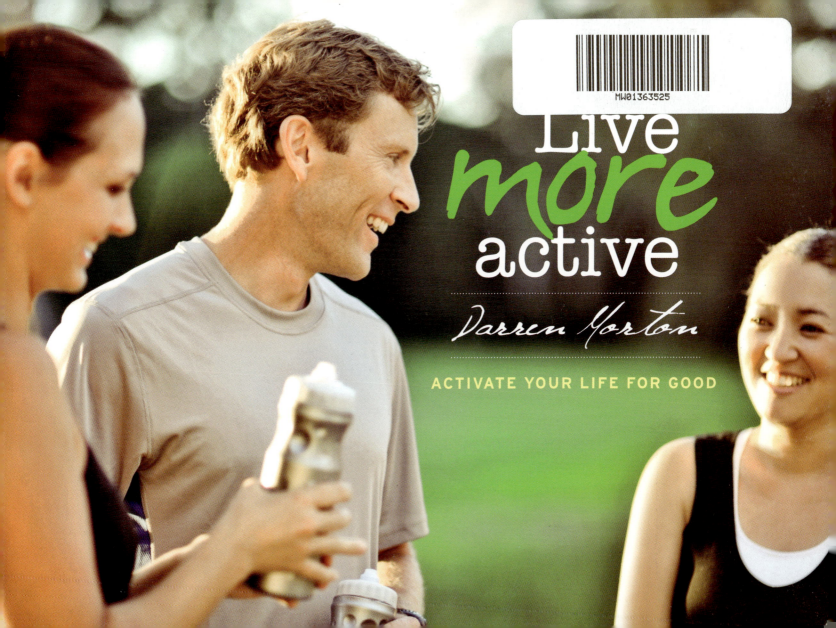

Copyright © Second edition, 2016, Darren Morton. All rights reserved.
First edition, 2014.

Medical Disclaimer: The ideas, concepts and opinions expressed in this work are intended to be used for educational purposes only. This work is sold and distributed with the understanding that the authors and publisher are not rendering medical advice of any kind, nor is this work intended to (a) replace competent and licensed professional medical advice from a physician to a patient, or (b) diagnose, prescribe or treat any disease, condition, illness or injury. Readers should seek the advice of their individual doctor prior to and during participation in these lifestyle activities. The author and publisher of this work disclaim any and all responsibility to any person or entity for any liability, loss or damage caused or alleged to be caused directly or indirectly as a result of the use, application or interpretation of the material in this work.

Complete Health Improvement Program (CHIP), CHIP Heart logo and Lifestyle Medicine Institute logo are trademarks of the Lifestyle Medicine Institute LLC. Used by permission. Graphics on pages 6, 13, 16 and 39 designed by Shane Winfield and used by permission of the Lifestyle Medicine Institute LLC.

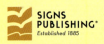 Proudly published and printed in Australia by
Signs Publishing Company, Warburton, Australia.

For more information or to purchase additional copies of this book, visit **www.DrDarrenMorton.com**

This Book Was
Edited by Nathan Brown
Proofread by Lindy Schneider and Nathan Brown
Designed by DEC Creatives (Dominique Cherry)
Cover design by DEC Creatives (Dominique Cherry)
Typeset in Interstate Light 9.5/13

ISBN 978 1 925044 44 7 (print)
ISBN 978 1 925044 45 4 (ebook)

FOREWORD

It's often been said that if exercise could be put into a pill it would be prescribed with great regularity and enthusiasm. Unfortunately, it requires some effort and there's little money to be made from its sale.

That doesn't detract from its effectiveness. As known by its exponents—but now also proven from research—it is not doing something unnatural that is healthy, but not doing something that is perfectly natural to human beings that makes us unhealthy.

A re-institution of that form of natural activity, which human beings have carried out as part of daily living for almost all our history has now been shown to be effective in preventing and even reducing the effects of the modern chronic diseases that now make up around 70 per cent of all reasons for visiting a doctor.

Two recent publications have reinforced this:

❯ The first study, by respected exercise researcher Dr Frank Booth and colleagues from the University of Missouri—entitled "Lack of exercise is a major cause of chronic disease"[1]—lists 35 chronic conditions for which physical activity has preventive benefits. The list includes some obvious conditions—such as heart disease, type 2 diabetes and stroke—but also some that may not seem that obvious, including erectile dysfunction, endometrial cancer and constipation. More importantly, Booth presents evidence of declines in both total and quality years of life with inactivity that make inactivity one of the most important causes of chronic disease known.

❯ A second article, by researchers at the London School of Economics and Political Science,[2] is an even more objective assessment of exercise as a treatment method in comparison with well-known prescription drugs. Comparing studies on exercise as a treatment for a range of problems such as blood pressure, stroke, type 2 diabetes and heart failure, with the most effective drugs usually prescribed for these problems, exercise was shown to have similar effects in terms of benefits in reduced mortality.

A problem in instituting these findings is that people seem to have forgotten—or never learned—how to exercise, because modern technology has taken daily activity away from us. And while there are countless books claiming to show you how to achieve magic benefits with minimum effort, few have a good scientific basis for their claims.

Darren Morton is one writer, teacher and researcher who knows his stuff. Not only this, but he knows how to get the message across, while being a good example of practising what he preaches. In *Live More: Active*, Morton gives clear, concise and entertaining advice on how to get the most from an exercise (and lifestyle) program. This is a useful and entertaining addition to our knowledge in the field.

Garry Egger

Professor of Health and Human Sciences, Southern Cross University
Author, National Physical Activity Guidelines (Australia)

1. F Booth, et al (2012), "Lack of exercise is a major cause of chronic disease," *Comprehensive Physiology*, Vol 2, pages 1143-1211.
2. H Naci and J Ioannidis (2013), "Comparative effectiveness of exercise and drug interventions on mortality outcomes: metaepidemiological study," *British Journal of Medicine*, Vol 347, f5577.

CONTENTS

Foreword　　　　　　*page* iii

Introduction　　　　　*page* 2

SECTION 1: Activate your life for good

Chapter 1	**SOS:** How to be saved from the inactivity crisis	*page* 6
Chapter 2	*Step 1:* **S**it less, move more!	*page* 12
Chapter 3	Discovering motivation	*page* 18
Chapter 4	*Step 2:* **O**xygenate	*page* 37
Chapter 5	Excuses, excuses!	*page* 51
Chapter 6	*Step 3:* **S**trengthen and stretch	*page* 64
Chapter 7	Moving to success	*page* 96
Chapter 8	The power of belief	*page* 112

SECTION 2: Your 21-day activation challenge　　*page* 123

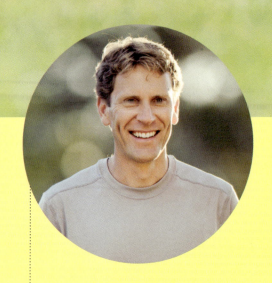

Introduction

Congratulations on picking up this book and opening it—your first active step toward living more!

There is no better time to activate your life than today and, throughout this book, I will provide you with everything I have learned during the past 25 years in health and fitness—as an exercise scientist, lecturer, researcher, athlete, coach and trainer—to give you the best possible chance of successfully activating your life in the long-term.

Experience has taught me that it is easy to get people moving in the short-term. We have all had bursts of enthusiasm that caused us to exercise—once. But sticking with it is the challenge. This is why this book is structured in two sections.

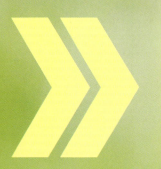

In **Section 1**, you will learn the latest *information* about exercise and active living—what to do and why. We will also clear up many of the "mistruths" about exercise that bombard us today. You will discover what the optimal active lifestyle looks like, and the ideal type and level of physical activity required to produce the best possible health outcomes. By the end of this book, you will know everything you need to know about exercise and being active.

But information alone isn't usually enough to produce long-term changes in what we do. Throughout the book, we will also explore the secrets of successful behavior change so you can activate your life for good. You will be pleased to know it has little to do with willpower.

Section 2 is where this book "comes alive." Over 21 days you get to put what you have learned into practice—to road test it. I can't stress enough the importance of engaging with Section 2 as it will take this book beyond just a good read to a potentially life-changing experience. It is where you truly discover the *will* and the *way* to live more active. Section 2 is so important you can start there, if you prefer, as it will keep referring you back to the relevant parts of Section 1 anyway.

I also strongly encourage you to team up with someone or a group of others to join you on the 21-day *Live More: Active* challenge. Having personal support can make a huge difference, so find a friend, rope in a spouse or rally a group of co-workers.

Whether your doctor has said you need to exercise more "or else," you want to shed some weight to feel better about yourself, or you just want more energy and vitality, this book can help you live more—both in quantity and quality.

It is a privilege to act as your guide on this life-enriching journey toward living more active. I am cheering you on! It won't take long before you begin to notice great changes—so make today count.

Choose to live your best life. Live more active!

To Dad,
for always supporting my efforts to live more active.

SECTION 1:

Activate your life for good

DAY 1

Chapter One

SOS: How to be saved from the inactivity crisis

We are facing an inactivity crisis. It has been estimated that people living in developed countries are on average 60 to 70 per cent less active than a century ago, which equates to walking about 10 miles (16 kilometers) less every day.[1]

Did that statistic sink in? This is a huge downturn in our activity levels—and most of it has occurred in the past 40 years. Even more alarming, it shows no sign of turning around. It is hardly surprising that it has been suggested physical inactivity may be the most important public health problem of the 21st Century.[2] "Physical inactivity now kills more people than smoking—about 5.3 million deaths globally are attributable to physical inactivity compared to 5.1 million for smoking."[3]

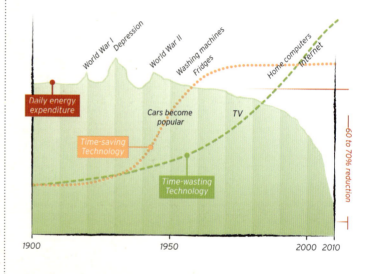

The changing patterns of physical activity in industrialized countries over the 20th Century.[4]

> *"Evidence supports the conclusion that physical inactivity is one of the most important health problems of the 21st Century, and may even be the most important."* – Professor Stephen Blair

This inactivity crisis presents such a health problem because we are *made to move*. The human body is designed to be active and things go wrong when it is not operated according to this design brief.

Many factors have contributed to the inactivity crisis, but the advent of "modern conveniences" is largely to blame. We have ingeniously created devices that allow us to expend less energy doing our daily tasks. They wash the dishes for us, deliver warm water straight to our bath so we don't have to walk or work to get it, lift us higher in a building by bypassing the stairs, and change the channel on our TV with the press of a remote button so we don't have to get out of our seat. It has been suggested that if the TV and refrigerator weren't so far apart, some of us would get no exercise at all. While these modern additions to our lifestyle are convenient, they have come at a huge cost to our activity levels—and our associated wellbeing. These innovative technologies have especially changed the nature of our work, transportation and recreation.

If the TV and refrigerator weren't so far apart, some of us would get no exercise at all!

› Work

In the 1950s, Dr Jerry Morris first documented the dangers of inactivity in a study of more than 30,000 London bus service employees.[5] According to Dr Morris, the bus drivers—who sat in their comfortable seats all day long—were about three times more likely to die from a heart attack than the conductors who were on their feet all day. Dr Morris also noted that the average uniform size of the drivers was larger than the uniforms of the conductors, suggesting a link between inactivity, obesity and heart health.

Since that time, most people's work has become less active. Even jobs that historically were extremely physically demanding have become more sedentary as machines have taken over. Especially during the past few decades, fewer and fewer people arrive at work on Monday morning anticipating a day of heavy physical labor. Instead, an increasing number sit in front of computer screens.

While work for many is becoming increasingly sedentary, retirement often exaggerates the inactivity problem.[6]

› Transportation

In years past, lengthy travel time was not a problem because it required us to use our legs. But today we get places by sitting—in the car, bus, train or plane. Furthermore, the length of time we spend in transportation has increased substantially with urbanization as an increasing number of individuals are forced to commute long distances to travel from the suburbs where they live to the city where they work. In large cities, it is not uncommon for individuals to travel two hours to work, then another two hours home. When added to the eight or more hours sitting at work, this represents a huge portion of the day spent inactive.

❯ Recreation

The invention of TV revolutionized the way people spent their free time, and the development of the internet and computer-based entertainment has further increased the time we are inactive. Indeed, "screen time" is a major contributor to our sedentary lifestyles. Unlike the 1950s when only about 10 per cent of homes had a television set,[7] today almost every home has at least one. Similarly, the number of homes with internet access has skyrocketed since the late 1990s.

Unfortunately, it is not only adults who are glued to screens: children are also spending far too much time playing video games, communicating with their friends over the internet or watching TV. Children are now often spending more than seven hours a day in front of a screen—TVs, computers, phones and other electronic devices—for entertainment.[8] Peak bodies such as the American Academy of Pediatrics encourage parents to limit their children's screen time to not more than two hours per day.[9]

Tips for getting your kids to unplug and play[10]

- *Make your child's bedroom a screen-free zone.*
- *Make family rules to reduce time spent using electronic entertainment and stick to them.*
- *Use a timer or an alarm clock to monitor time spent using electronic entertainment.*
- *Set certain times when your child is not allowed to use electronic entertainment, such as during daylight hours, and before and after school.*
- *Limit the number of TVs, electronic game consoles and computers you have in your home.*
- *Be a role model: limit the time you spend using electronic entertainment and be active.*
- *Provide active play opportunities for your child.*
- *Talk with other parents about ideas for getting your child to unplug and play.*
- *Don't rely on movement-based video games as a substitute for active play.*

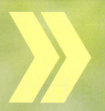

Rescue from the inactivity crisis—SOS

To be saved from the inactivity crisis, we need to apply SOS. SOS sums up the three steps to the optimal active lifestyle, which represents the ideal level and type of activity you should perform to beat the inactivity crisis and experience amazing benefits.

During the next 21 days, we will examine these three steps in detail, but here is a snapshot:

STEP 1: *Sit less, move more.*

We start by exploring the emerging evidence that too much "sit time" is not good for us, then consider strategies for breaking up prolonged periods of sitting. You will also be introduced to the pedometer—or step counter—a useful tool for monitoring how much you move throughout the day, as well as motivating you to get out of your seat and on your feet more often. If you don't already have a pedometer, you need to race out and buy one—they are not expensive.

If you have a smart phone, you can also download pedometer apps for free. One of my favorites is "Pacer" because it also reminds you when you haven't moved in a while.

STEP 2: *Oxygenate.*

Next we examine the life-giving properties of oxygen and the best way to deliver it to the tissues of your body that crave it for health and healing—aerobic physical activity. By the way, this is not where it gets hard! At no point on this journey toward the optimal active lifestyle are you going to be asked to pound the pavement in a lather of sweat with your tongue hanging out while clutching your chest, so relax. I am fully aware that one of the main reasons two-thirds of adults fail to embrace an adequately active lifestyle is because they don't like exercise.[11] Many of us associate exercise with pain and sweat, neither of which are endearing qualities. Fortunately, the old adage—"No pain, no gain"—doesn't stack up in light of the most recent studies showing exercise need not be exhausting to produce great benefits. This journey need not be painful! You don't have to endure it; you are meant to enjoy it.

STEP 3: **Strengthen and stretch.**

Finally, we focus on our muscles and how to make them strong and supple. Again, you are not going to be required to do anything too taxing—no grunting noises required! And you don't have to join a gym. You can be your own gym with simple strengthening and stretching exercises you can perform in your own home.

If you think strengthening and stretching exercises are not necessary for you, you are wrong. Everyone can benefit tremendously from these exercises, especially older females, and this is why such exercises form an integral component of the optimal active lifestyle. To make these exercises easier for you, I have included a DVD in the back of this book to guide you through.

In addition to learning the three steps toward the optimal active lifestyle, we will also explore the secrets and strategies for successfully following through and making them part of your long-term lifestyle. We will examine what drives your behaviors and how to harness this force to discover motivation that doesn't rely on willpower. We will consider the common barriers people face to being active—which often masquerade as excuses—and how to remove them.

We will also explore strategies for setting yourself up to be successful, which involve knowing yourself and what works best for you, as well as how to negotiate living in an environment where inactivity is the default. Finally, we will focus on how what we believe about ourselves can shape our patterns of living, for better or worse.

Chapter One References

[1] N Vogels, et al (2004), "Estimating Changes in Daily Physical Activity Levels over Time: Implication for Health Interventions from a Novel Approach," *International Journal of Sports Medicine*, Vol 25, pages 607-10.

[2] S Blair (2009), "Physical inactivity: the biggest public health problem of the 21st century," *British Journal of Sports Medicine*, Vol 43 No 1, pages 1-2.

[3] C Wen and X Wu (2012), "Stressing harms of physical inactivity to promote exercise," *Lancet*, Vol 38, pages 192-3.

[4] Vogels, op cit.

[5] J N Morris, et al (1953), "Coronary heart disease and physical activity of work," *The Lancet*, Vol 2, pages 1111-20.

[6] U Berger, et al (2005), "The impact of retirement on physical activity," *Ageing & Society,* Vol 25, pages 181-95.

[7] R C Brownson, T K Boehmer and D A Luke (2005), "Declining rate of physical activity in the US: what are the contributors?" *Annual Review of Public Health*, Vol 26, pages 421-43.

[8] American Academy of Pediatrics (2010), "AAP Updates Guidance to Help Families Make Positive Media Choices." <http://www.aap.org/en-us/about-the-aap/aap-press-room/Pages/AAP-Updates-Guidance-to-Help-Families-Make-Positive-Media-Choices.aspx>.

[9] ibid.

[10] Heart Foundation, <https://www.heartfoundation.org.au/SiteCollectionDocuments/Healthy%20Kids%20-%20Previous%20Unplug%20+%20Play%20Campaign%20Brochure.pdf>.

[11] Australian Bureau of Statistics (2008), National Health Survey. <http://www.abs.gov.au/ausstats/abs@.nsf/Lookup/4835.0.55.001main+features32007-08>.

Chapter Two

Step 1: Sit less, move more!

Most of us are naturals when it comes to sitting—we perform it effortlessly. Of course, the reason is that it is effortless, and therein lies the problem. We are made to move, but we are spending more time "bottom-dwelling" than ever.

Alarmingly, researchers are discovering that the long-term ill-health consequences of too much sitting—and not enough moving—are distinct from the consequences of not exercising. In other words, while exercising daily has many health-promoting benefits, if you spend the rest of your day sitting around and not moving, your risk of ill-health, disease and premature death jumps back up!

Study 1: In a study of more than 120,000 adults monitored for 14 years, people who sat for extended periods in their leisure time and did not exercise had a greatly increased risk of premature death—a 94 per cent increase for women and a 48 per cent increase for men. At first there appeared to be nothing surprising about these results, as it simply demonstrated the well-established importance of being physically active for good health. But as the researchers mined the data more thoroughly, they noticed a fascinating trend. Those individuals who exercised regularly but then sat for extended periods during the day still had a greatly increased death rate—as much as a 40 per cent higher rate for women and 20 per cent for men.[1]

Study 2: In another study, after the researchers took into account most of the recognized risk factors for disease, such as whether an individual smoked, had high blood pressure or a long-standing illness, was obese, socially disadvantaged or even physically active, those individuals who engaged in more than four hours of screen-based entertainment per day had a 48 per cent increased chance of dying from all causes and a 125 per cent increased likelihood of suffering a heart attack or stroke.[2]

ACCUMULATED SIT TIME OF AN "ACTIVE COUCH POTATO"[3]

- SLEEP 8 hours
- WATCHING TV, READING 4 hours
- EAT DINNER 30 minutes
- DRIVE HOME 1 hour
- WORK ON COMPUTER 4 hours
- LUNCH 30 minutes
- WORK ON COMPUTER 4 hours
- DRIVE TO WORK 1 hour
- BRISK WALK 30 minutes
- STRENGTH TRAINING 30 minutes

It seems "taking a seat" has never been so hazardous! The problem is that we live in a society in which sitting is the default. As pictured, it is easy to accumulate 15 hours of sit time in a day, despite this individual being diligent enough to perform 60 minutes of exercise, which is far beyond the achievements of most of us! Such individuals are often described as "*active* couch potatoes."

Inactivity physiology

The dangers of prolonged sitting are becoming so apparent that a new field of study—"inactivity physiology"—is emerging. Researchers in this field have discovered that prolonged periods of sitting and not moving alter the body's control over cholesterol in a negative way—especially the bad "LDL" cholesterol—and places individuals at increased risk of cardiovascular disease.[4]

But it is not only the amount of sedentary time we accumulate; it is how it is accumulated. Prolonged *uninterrupted* sit time appears to be the real danger, providing us with some hope. Regularly breaking up periods of sitting with short periods of movement—even just standing for a few minutes every half hour or so—is associated with a slimmer waist, lower body weight, less fat in the blood and lower blood-sugar levels.[5]

Live More **ACTIVE** | 13

The take-away message: Most of us are sitting far too much in an uninterrupted fashion—and it is to our detriment. The solution? Sit less and move more!

No longer can we afford to think of having to move as a time-wasting bother. Instead, we need to start thinking of it as an opportunity to invest in our own health and wellbeing. This change in mind-set is critical. In fact, the Australian Physical Activity Guidelines insightfully begin with, "Think of movement as an opportunity, not an inconvenience."[6]

Every bit of movement counts—and your journey toward the optimal active lifestyle starts with sitting less and moving more. The old proverb was right: "The journey of a thousand miles begins with a single step."

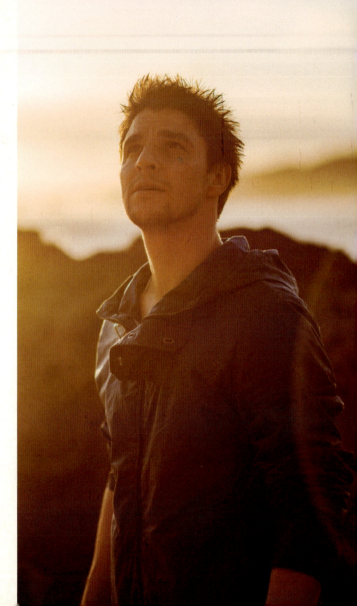

PRACTICAL TIPS FOR SITTING LESS[7]

At home

- Move around the house when talking on the telephone.
- Take the batteries out of the TV remote control so you have to get out of your seat to change channels.
- Stand up and walk around the house during TV commercial breaks.
- Do household chores that involve standing, such as ironing, while watching TV.
- Stand to read the morning newspaper.

At work

- Stand and take a break from your computer every 30 minutes.
- Stand periodically during long meetings. (Explain what you are doing at the start and you might encourage others to do likewise.)
- Stand to greet a visitor to your worksite.
- Stand during phone calls.
- Take the stairs.
- Drink more water so that you have to go fetch it and visit the bathroom more often.
- Move items such as your trash can, filing cabinet and printer further away, so you are forced to get out of your seat to use them.
- Use a height-adjustable desk, so you can alternate between sitting and standing.
- Organize standing or "walk while we talk" meetings instead of the usual sit-a-thons. Your brain will work better, too!
- Stand at the back of the room during presentations.
- Eat your lunch away from your desk.

When travelling

- Park your car further away from your destination and walk the rest of the way.
- Plan regular breaks during long car trips.
- Use public transport so you have to walk to and from stops or stations.
- Get on or off public transport one stop or station before your destination and walk the rest of the way.
- On public transport, offer your seat to someone who needs it.

DAY 3

"I was going to walk today, but my toes voted against me 10 to 1."

› Step it out. A useful device for keeping track of how much you are moving throughout the day, as well as providing motivation to get out of your seat more often, is a pedometer—or step counter. For best results, clip your pedometer to your hip above your right knee, although on your shoes can work well, too.

In recent years, electronic wristbands that sync with your smartphone have become increasingly popular. Not only do these count steps, these devices also monitor other physiological markers of activity, fitness and wellbeing. This information can be helpful on your journey to more active living, but these devices tend to be considerably more expensive than a simple pedometer.

So how many steps a day should you aim for? The commonly cited goal is to achieve 10,000 steps per day. This number was first proposed back in the 1960s in Japan where walking clubs embraced the nickname "manpo-kei" given to pedometers by the manufacturers, which literally means "10,000 steps meter."[8]

Activity level

Classification of activity level according to daily steps achieved[9]

Number of steps per day

LESS THAN 5000
SEDENTARY

5000-7499
LOW ACTIVE

7500-9999
SOMEWHAT ACTIVE

10,000-12,500
ACTIVE

MORE THAN 12,500
HIGHLY ACTIVE

As shown, individuals who achieve 10,000 steps per day are considered "active." The number of daily steps recommended for children is 13,000 for boys and 11,000 for girls.[10] Older adults, or those with chronic diseases like heart disease, might need to set themselves a slightly lower target.

While pedometers have some limitations—they don't measure the *type* of steps you take, nor do they count any of the steps you take if you forget to wear them—they can be extremely motivational. When you wear a pedometer, there is a tendency to keep checking it and this self-monitoring can cause you to move more. People will commonly take an extra 2000 steps per day when wearing a pedometer,[11] which in one study of low-activity individuals resulted in a reduction of about 1 inch (2.5 centimeters) in waist circumference.[12] Pedometers can also be educational as they can show you how making relatively small excursions, like regularly getting out of your chair to fill your water bottle, increases your daily step tally. This highlights the value of "incidental activity."

› Step up. The first step toward the optimal active lifestyle is literally a step, leading to less bottom-dwelling and more moving. As pedometers are such useful devices for monitoring how we are moving, your challenge for this week involves counting steps, so turn to Section 2 and step up! And while you put Step 1 into practice over the next week, let's turn our attention to the critical issue of how to discover motivation.

Chapter Two References

1. A Patel, et al (2010), "Leisure Time Spent Sitting in Relation to Total Mortality in a Prospective Cohort of US Adults," *American Journal of Epidemiology*, Vol 172, pages 419-29.

2. E Stamatakis, et al (2011), "Screen-Based Entertainment Time, All-Cause Mortality, and Cardiovascular Events: Population-Based Study With Ongoing Mortality and Hospital Events Follow-Up," *Journal of the American College of Cardiology*, Vol 57, pages 292-9.

3. National Heart Foundation of Australia (2011), "Sitting less for adults," <www.heartfoundation.org.au/SiteCollectionDocuments/HW-PA-SittingLess-Adults.pdf>.

4. M Hamilton, et al (2008), "Too Little Exercise and Too Much Sitting: Inactivity Physiology and the Need for New Recommendations on Sedentary Behavior," *Current Cardiovascular Risk Reports*, Vol 2, pages 292-8.

5. G N Healy, et al (2008), "Breaks in sedentary time—beneficial associations with metabolic risk," *Diabetes Care*, Vol 31 No 4, pages 661-6.

6. Department of Health and Aging (2005). <http://www.health.gov.au/internet/main/publishing.nsf/content/health-pubhlth-strateg-phys-act-guidelines#guidelines_adults>.

7. Adapted from National Heart Foundation of Australia, 2011.

8. C Tudor-Locke, et al (2008). "Revisiting 'how many steps are enough?'" *Medicine and Science in Sports and Exercise*, Vol 40 No 7 supplement, pages S537-43.

9. ibid.

10. S Vincent, R P Pangrazi, et al (2003), "Activity Levels and body mass index of children in the United States, Sweden and Australia," *Medicine and Science in Sport and Exercise*, Vol 35 No 8, pages 1367-73.

11. D M Bravata et al (2007). "Using Pedometers to Increase Physical Activity and Improve Health: A Systematic Review," *Journal of the American Medical Association*, Vol 298 No 19, pages 2296-304.

12. T Dwyer, et al (2007), "The inverse relationship between number of steps per day and obesity in a population-based sample—the AusDiab study," *International Journal of Obesity*, Vol 31, pages 797-804.

DAY 4

Chapter Three
Discovering motivation

Thousands of years ago, Aristotle came up with the idea that we humans are primarily motivated by pleasure and pain—we do things to *achieve* pleasure and we do things to *avoid* pain. It's all about the carrot and the stick!

To state it simply, we do what we do for a feeling—and there is a good explanation for this. Neurophysiologists, who study how the brain is put together and works, have discovered that the part of our brain responsible for our emotions (or feelings) is the same part primarily responsible for our drives.[1] It is referred to as the Limbic System.

This explains why strong feelings excite our best efforts—take love and fear as examples—whereas when we lack feelings, we are apathetic, unmotivated and uninspired to action. For proof, ask a couch potato why they don't get up and do some exercise and they will tell you quite frankly it's because they don't *feel* like it!

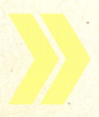

Get a taste for it! The Limbic System—our emotional brain—is highly stimulated by smell and taste.[2] This explains in part why people "comfort eat." Essentially, when our Limbic System gets emotionally down or stressed and it wants a pick-me-up, it drives us to eat. Unfortunately, it tends to drive us to eat sweet and fatty foods that are not helpful when it comes to optimizing our health! As Dr Neal Barnard points out, no-one says, "I feel so upset that I feel like eating a whole head of broccoli!"[3]

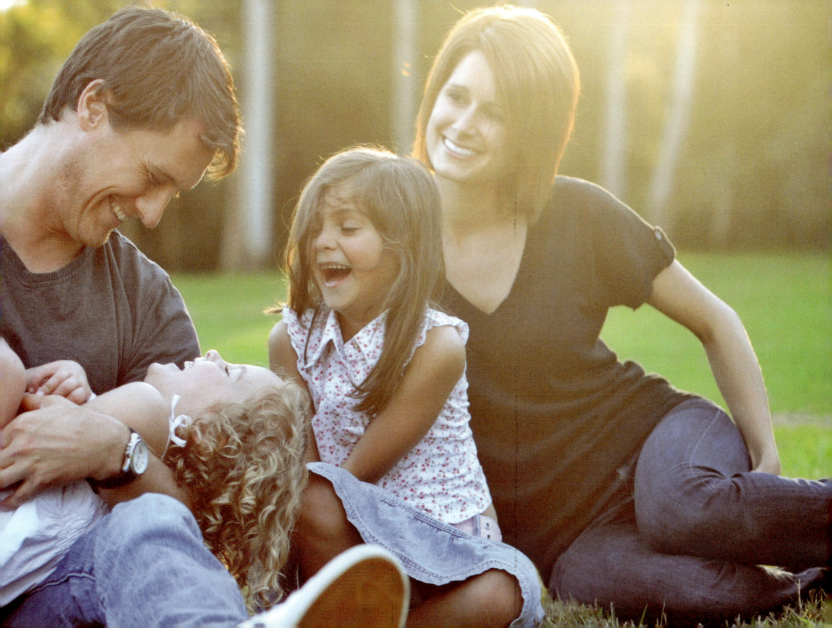

What this means: To discover motivation and hold on to it, you need to get emotional about it. It is no surprise that the word "emotion" literally means "to move." To successfully follow through in the long-term, whether it be with a more active lifestyle or any other behavior change, you need to feel strongly about it. Willpower alone won't get you there.

Story: Kevin used to scoff at those "crazy people" who punished themselves with daily exercise. That all changed when Kevin was 31, after his heart attack. As he lay on the floor clutching his chest, intense pain radiating down his arm and up his neck, Kevin thought he was about to die. The experience terrified him. Fortunately, Kevin survived and when his cardiologist told him that one of the best things he could do to aid his recovery and avoid it happening again was to become active, he was ready to listen. Today, Kevin is only half the man he used to be—he has lost that much weight—and has morphed into one of those "crazy people" who doesn't miss a day without being physically active. Pain can be a powerful motivator.

Using willpower you might be able to force yourself to go walking a few times, but chances are you will give up. This is because willpower arises from the thinking part of your brain—the cerebral cortex. As thoughts can be fickle, so too is our willpower. Has your thinking brain ever come up with a good reason why you *shouldn't* exercise, even though you had decided to become more active only a few days earlier?

But feelings are more enduring. Strong feelings can drive behaviors for years. In order to discover long-lasting motivation, you therefore need to move beyond *thinking* you should to *feeling* you must. The first step to achieving this involves identifying really good, emotive reasons for adopting your desired new behavior—reasons that involve pleasure and pain.

The benefits of living more active

Consider the perils of the sedentary lifestyle—the pain you can expect if you are not active—and the benefits of living more active—the pleasure that will come from following through and moving more. As you will see, activating your life can enable you to live longer, leaner and livelier. In Section 2, you will reflect on how these facts make you *feel*.

› LIVE LONGER

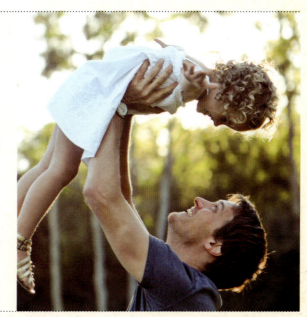

Inactivity increases your risk of dying young, whereas being physically active extends your life. More than 30 years ago, it was first observed that champion male Finnish skiers lived on average 4.1 years longer than "average" Finnish men.[4] Since that time, it has become clear that former elite athletes do tend to live longer than us mere mortals,[5] but you don't have to be an Olympian to look forward to a long life.

An investigation of the longest-living people on earth—the Okinawans, Sardinians and Seventh-day Adventists—showed one of the things they all had in common is they "moved naturally."[6] In other words, they engaged in plenty of physical activity as part of their daily living.

A concentrated study of the Seventh-day Adventist community—the famous "Adventist Health Study"—identified being physically active as one of five key lifestyle choices for increasing your lifespan. This research found that being physically active, along with not smoking, eating nuts regularly, being vegetarian, and maintaining a healthy body weight, could add as many as 10 years to your life, with each of these recommended lifestyle choices adding between 1.5 and 2.5 years.[7]

A long-term follow-up study of more than 50,000 men and women in the renowned Aerobics Center Longitudinal Study showed just how important fitness level is in preventing premature death.[8]

As shown on this graph, the percentage of deaths attributable to low fitness level was much greater than the other conditions listed, apart from high blood pressure in males. Low fitness level was about twice as dangerous as smoking! Other studies have also shown low cardio-respiratory fitness to be more predictive of premature death than smoking.[9]
Further research also specifically links inactivity with cancer risk: "Physical inactivity is the second greatest contributor, behind tobacco smoking, to the cancer burden in Australia."[10]

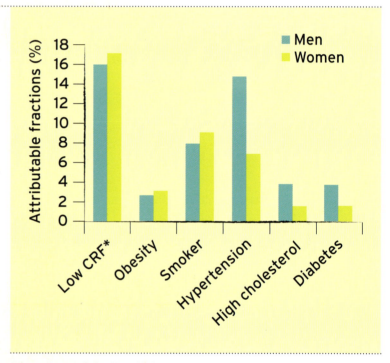

Percentage of deaths attributable to low cardio-respiratory fitness, obesity, smoking, hypertension (high blood pressure), high cholesterol and diabetes.[11]

Another recent study from the same researchers showed that being fit in your middle-age years (the average age of the participants in their study was 49 years) resulted in less years of being unwell in the later stages of life—a desirable state referred to as "morbidity compression."[12] This shows that fitter people remain healthy for a greater portion of their longer lives. Who doesn't want that!

So why does being physically active enable us to live longer? One of the key reasons is because it offers protection against many common but undesirable conditions, including:[13]

› Coronary heart disease	› Stroke	› High blood pressure
› High cholesterol	› Type 2 diabetes	› Lung cancer
› Colon cancer	› Breast cancer	› Endometrial cancer
› Erectile dysfunction	› Constipation	

In fact, inactivity is now linked to 35 chronic conditions, which in addition to those already listed above, include osteoporsis, chronic pain and depression.[14]

But while being physically active can help *prevent* these conditions, it can also help *manage* and, in some cases, even *treat* them.

For heart disease

In 1968, when Dr Kenneth Cooper wrote his pioneering book *The Aerobics Revolution*, which promoted the benefits of regular physical exercise, his ideas went against the thinking of the medical establishment. At the time, if a person suffered a heart attack, they were prescribed bed rest and told to never exercise again. Today we know this is the worst advice possible. In patients with stable coronary heart disease, it has been found that those who adopt an exercise program have better survival rates than those who have stents surgically inserted in their narrowed blood vessels.[15]

For high blood pressure and high cholesterol

For those with high cholesterol levels and elevated blood pressure, regular exercise performed right is also excellent. In people with hypertension (high blood pressure), just a single bout of exercise will usually decrease their blood pressure by about 5-7 mmHg for about one day afterward.[16] I consistently observe this in my research on the lifestyle modification program referred to as CHIP—the Complete Health Improvement Program. CHIP is brilliant at bringing down "bad" cholesterol levels within just 30 days.[17] While CHIP is a comprehensive program that addresses all aspects of wellbeing—diet, physical activity, stress, rest, emotional wellbeing, etc—findings of one of my graduate students show that increasing physical activity levels is independently associated with improvements in all health measures, including cholesterol, blood pressure, body weight and blood sugar levels.[18]

For diabetes

Exercise has been described by the American Dietetic Association as a "cornerstone" in the management of diabetes.[19] Exercise makes insulin work more effectively and therefore assists with blood sugar control—a single bout of aerobic exercise can makes insulin work better for up to three days.[20] Performing regular resistance exercises, like those introduced later in this book, have also been shown to produce positive improvements in blood sugar control that match and sometimes exceed that typically produced by conventional drug treatments.[21] However, it is important that people with diabetes take special care of their feet during exercise and pay particular attention to their blood sugar level.

Other benefits

There are many more reasons why regular exercise is so good for us—it even increases fertility in women[22]—and some of the mechanisms are still only just beginning to be understood. Besides reducing "bad" cholesterol and increasing "good" cholesterol,[23] decreasing blood pressure and "flushing" the body of toxins, regular exercise increases the production of *antioxidants* in the body that neutralize damaging agents called free radicals.[24] Free radicals are known to contribute to the progression of many diseases—even the ageing process—so the fact that regular exercise can fight them is great. Moderate physical activity is also known to have anti-inflammatory properties and even boost the body's immune system.[25]

As has been said before, if you could develop a pill that packaged the benefits that come from regular physical activity, it would be a major medical breakthrough—you would get rich quick as everyone would want to swallow it. Exercise has been shown to be as effective as drug therapies, in terms of preventing death, for heart disease, rehabilitation after stroke, treatment of heart failure and prevention of diabetes. It is little wonder it can help us live longer.[26] The great news is that everyone can take this "pill"—and it's free! Appropriately, many peak exercise bodies including the American College of Sports Medicine and Exercise and Sports Science Australia have adopted the catch cry, "Exercise is medicine."

❯ LIVE LIVELIER

The oft-repeated quip about healthy living asks, "If I make positive lifestyle changes and kick the bad habits, will I live longer—or will it just feel longer?" Living longer is not so enticing if you constantly feel miserable. But while regular physical activity can add years to your life, it also adds life to your years—and it does this in two significant ways:

1. Energy boost

Regular exercise boosts your energy levels. When I teach undergraduate students about energy metabolism, I love to start by showing them a large poster covered with tiny writing that details the complex chemical pathways within the body involved in generating energy. Harnessing energy from an apple is no simple feat!

What is more amazing is to learn that when we challenge those metabolic pathways by asking them to speed up and generate energy more rapidly,

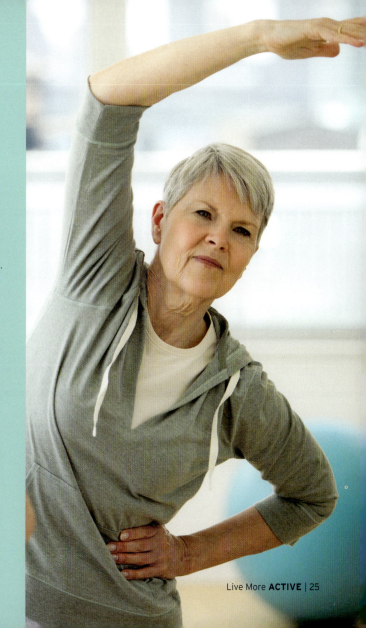

they respond by boosting the concentrations of key chemicals and increasing the activity of the enzymes that cause the metabolic mill to turn. So when we are regularly expending energy—by being physically active—we get more of it.

The body has three systems for generating energy, designed for short explosive bursts, medium efforts and the long-term grind. With the right kind of activity, the power and capacity of each one of these energy systems can be expanded. Athletes can have energetic capacities twice the size of sedentary people!

Having more available energy can improve many aspects of your life. One study found that when workers decreased their work hours and instead engaged in exercise, their productivity went up.[27] If you want more of the precious commodity that is "energy," exercise is the way to discover it.

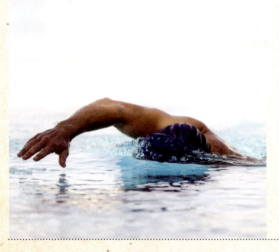

2. Mood upswing

Exercise is one of the best things you can do to lift your spirits—it has been referred to as the most under-utilized antidepressant. According to researchers, people who engage in exercise programs display fewer depressive symptoms and are less likely to develop major depressive disorders.[28] And for those with major depression, the effectiveness of exercise seems to be generally comparable to antidepressant medication, psychotherapy and cognitive therapy.[29] (Note: Medications should only be adjusted in consultation with your doctor.) Clearly, exercise can have a positive effect not only on your body, but on your brain as well, and there are many potential explanations.

Exercise increases blood flow to the brain.
As organs of the body function best with a good blood supply, there is increasing evidence that the increased blood flow to the brain during exercise enhances cognitive and brain function.[30] It is hardly surprising that many of the great scholars of the ancient world, including Aristotle, walked with their students as they taught. In fact, the school of philosophy in Ancient Greece founded by Aristotle was called the "Peripatetic school," which translates as "given to walking about." Personally, I find all my best ideas come to me while I am running!

Studies among older individuals have shown that regular physical activity decreases mental decline, protects against a decrease in brain size that often accompanies ageing, and enhances learning and memory—improvements in learning can occur after just one week of exercise.[31]

Proprioceptors are stimulated. Distributed throughout your body are many nerves endings called proprioceptors. Proprioceptors are specialized sensory nerve endings found in muscles, tendons and joints that relay information to your brain about your body position and movement.[32] When these proprioceptors are dynamically activated, as occurs during exercise, they flood the brain with stimulating messages. One part of the brain that is tremendously influenced by the messages proprioceptors send is the Limbic System, which as we have already learnt, is responsible for our emotional state.[33] Hence, "motion creates emotion" and dynamic exercise can make us feel better.

Endorphins are released in the brain. Exercise can stimulate the release of mood-enhancing chemicals—called endorphins—in your brain, especially when the exercise is intense.[34] Incredibly, endorphins have similar effects to opiate drugs in that they reduce pain and make you feel euphoric—they are responsible for the "high" runners often report and explain why regular exercisers find such pleasure in their daily "fix."[35] Unlike opiate drugs, however, they are good for you!

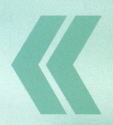

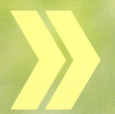

Sleep habits improve with exercise.

Being physically active can make you feel more alive by improving your sleep habits. Living in a constant state of sleep deprivation as a result of poor-quality sleep will make anyone feel lousy—and those who have to live with them! Insomnia and subsequent daytime tiredness affects many individuals but physical activity can burn up the stress hormones that keep us awake at night.[36]

So many of us live frantic lives that activate the body's "fight or flight" response designed to gear our bodies up to do something *physical*—either start throwing punches to defend ourselves or run like something is chasing us. When we do neither, we can find ourselves lying awake staring at the ceiling. Expending energy during the day by engaging in physical activity can help calm us down for a restful night's sleep. Early in the day is the best time to exercise if you suffer insomnia, so you have plenty of time to "come down" from the stress-relieving activity. Being active in the morning also helps set your body clock to daytime.

Feel good about yourself.

Regular physical activity can help you not only feel good in yourself, it can also help you feel good *about* yourself. Studies have shown that regular physical activity improves a person's perception of their physical condition and body attractiveness, and increases their sense of physical self-worth and overall self-esteem.[37] The same observation has been made among children, with higher levels of fitness offering a protective buffer to body-image concerns.[38] Feeling good about yourself and how you look is probably one of the most powerful motivators to be physically active for most people—call it vanity, but it really is a powerful driver. Importantly, it is not how we look that matters most, but how we feel about how we look that really counts. Regular exercise helps with both.

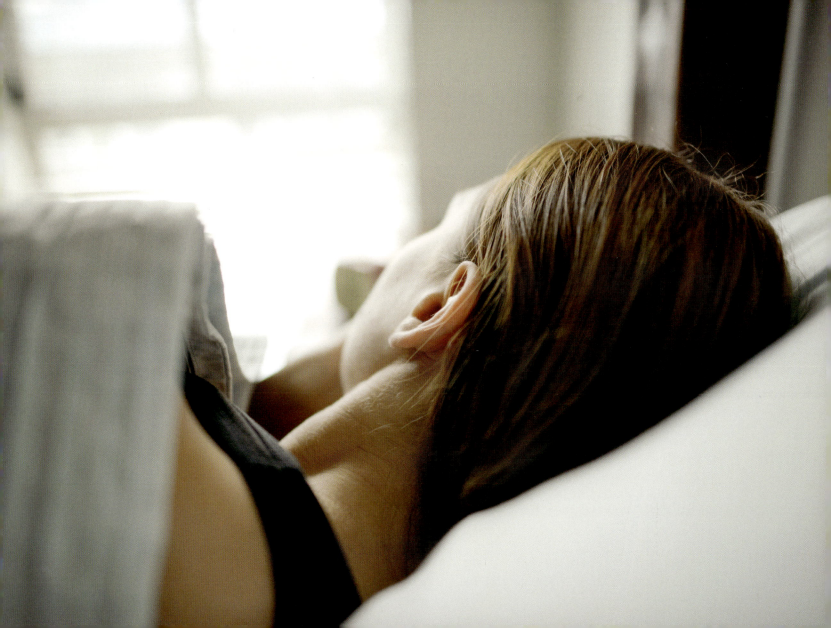

DAY 6

›LIVE LEANER

Worldwide, obesity has more than doubled since 1980, and today 65 per cent of the world's population live in countries where more people die as a result of being overweight than being underweight.[39] While genetics are often blamed for the obesity epidemic, genetics clearly don't explain the overwhelming increase in obesity over the past 30 years. The human genome has not changed significantly in that time!

DNA is not your destiny.

It is easy to be demotivated by the thought, "I have bad genes." But studies indicate that genetics only contribute about 30 per cent to our health outcomes—the bigger contributor (70 per cent) is lifestyle.[40] A fascinating field of research called *epigenetics* is showing that even if we have genes that predispose us to certain conditions and diseases, these genes are only "switched on" when exposed to certain lifestyle practices.[41] So the good news is that our genes need not be our fate. The new way of thinking is that, "Our genes load the gun, but our lifestyle pulls the trigger."

Defining overweight and obese.

Body Mass Index (BMI) is commonly used to determine overweight and obesity. BMI is calculated as:

Imperial:
BMI = Weight (pounds) / Height^2 (inches) x 703

Metric:
BMI = Weight (kilograms) / Height^2 (meters)

A BMI greater than 25 is considered "overweight" and above 30 "obese." Clearly the use of BMI has limitations—for example a muscular lean male can have a high BMI because muscle weighs more than fat—but it is helpful for population studies.

> Another helpful measure is waist girth. As fat in the abdominal area is more dangerous than fat in other places on the body such as the hips and thighs, waist circumference is better than BMI as a predictor of obesity-related health risk such as heart disease and diabetes.[42] Males should have a waist girth (measured level with the umbilicus without sucking in!) of less than 40 inches (102 centimeters), while females should be less than 35 inches (88 centimeters).

Numerous studies point to regular physical activity being an integral part of the solution to the obesity epidemic, especially for keeping lost weight off.[43] An expert report by the World Cancer Research Fund gave their highest commendation—"convincing"—to the role exercise plays in managing obesity.[44] Interestingly, the expert panel only judged the link between obesity and poor diet as "probable," which was the second-highest commendation. This is not to discount the importance of diet in effective weight management, but it does highlight that physical activity is, in the words of the expert panel, "of paramount importance."[45]

One reason exercise can be more effective than dieting for long-term weight loss is because once we get in the habit of it, we crave it. This occurs because the endorphins produced in response to exercise can be addictive—in a good way—and even cause regular exercisers to experience withdrawal-type symptoms—feeling antsy and irritable—if they can't be active.[46] So exercise can become a self-perpetuating behavior. By contrast, we never lose the desire to want to eat—hunger is a deeply ingrained, innate drive that prevents us from starving to death. It is almost impossible to go through life hungry, which is why calorie-restrictive diets are unsustainable in the long-term.

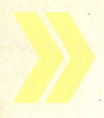

Exercise and appetite.

Does exercise increase appetite and therefore cause you to eat more? The answer seems to be both "yes" and "no."

Exercise does seem to increase appetite in people with a healthy weight. This is hardly surprising given that someone who is not carrying extra energy reserves—also known as body fat—needs to replace the energy used during exercise. However, exercise doesn't seem to cause the same increase in appetite in overweight individuals—it can actually decrease their feelings of hunger.[47]

Essentially, exercise seems to help with appetite regulation. It helps our brain get better at deciding how much energy our body actually needs, then adjusts our desire to eat accordingly.[48]

The importance of physical activity for long-term weight loss is highlighted by the findings of the National Weight Control Registry, which studies more than 10,000 individuals who have lost around 66 pounds (30 kilograms) and have kept it off for longer than five years.[49] The researchers have discovered four key things these success stories tend to have in common, and engaging in daily exercise is one of them. The other strategies include: eating foods of low energy density and prioritizing a hearty breakfast, weighing themselves regularly to self-monitor, and watching less than 10 hours of TV each week.

The take-away message: Exercise is vital for long-term weight loss.[50]

Activating your life can help you live longer, livelier and leaner. In Section 2, we explore what these benefits mean for *you*, so be sure to engage with this section now to maximize motivation.

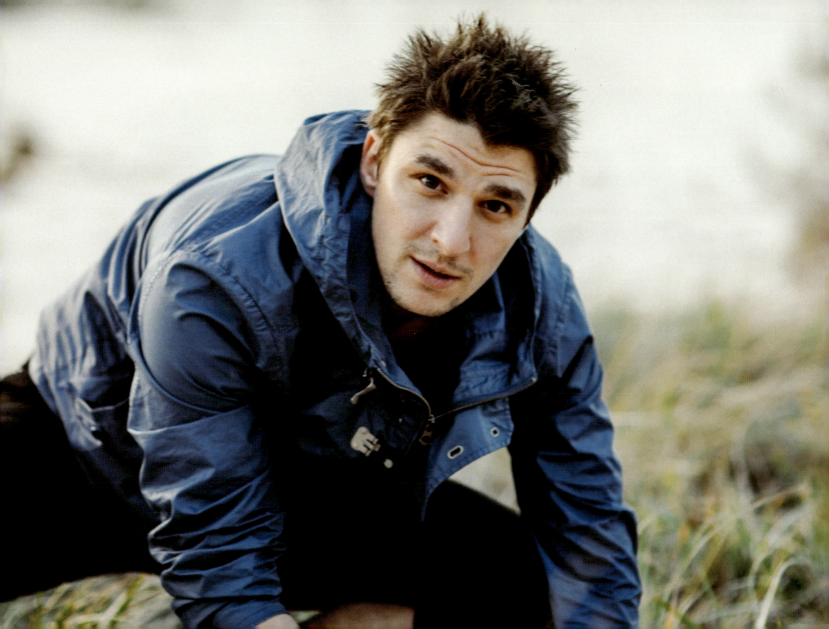

DAY 7

REST

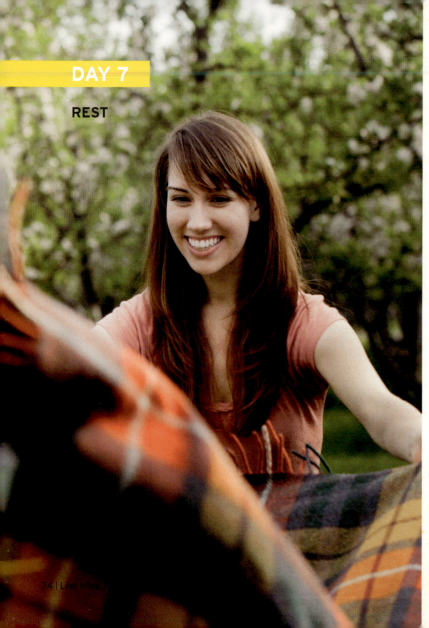

Chapter Three References

1. D L Clark, et al (2010), *The Brain and Behavior* (3rd edition), Cambridge University Press.

2. ibid.

3. N Barnard (2003), *Breaking the Food Seduction: The Hidden Reasons Behind Food Cravings—And 7 Steps to End Them Naturally*, St Martins Griffin.

4. M J Karvonen (1976), "Sports and Longevity," *Advances in Cardiology*, Vol 18, pages 243-8.

5. M Teramoto (2010), "Review: Mortality and longevity of elite athletes," *Journal of Science and Medicine in Sport*, Vol 13, pages 410-416.

6. D Buettner (2008), *The Blue Zone: Lessons for living longer from the people who have lived the longest*, National Geographic Society, Washington, page 231.

7. G E Fraser and D J Shavlik (2001), "Ten years of life: is it a matter of choice?" *Archive of Internal Medicine*, Vol 161, pages 1645-52.

8. S Blair (2009), "Physical inactivity: the biggest public health problem of the 21st century," *British Journal of Sports Medicine*, Vol 43 No 1, pages 1-2.

9. M Wei, et al (1999), "Relationship Between Low Cardiorespiratory Fitness and Mortality in Normal-Weight, Overweight, and Obese Men," *Journal of the American Medical Association*, Vol 282 No 16, pages 1547-53.

10. Department of Health (2014), "Research and Statistics," <www.health.gov.au/internet/main/publishing.nsf/Content/health-pubhlth-strateg-active-evidence.htm>.

11. Blair, op cit.

12. B L Willis, et al. (2012), "Midlife Fitness and the Development of Chronic Conditions in Later Life," *Archive of Internal Medicine*, Vol 172 No 17, pages 1333-40.

13. 2008 Physical Activity Guidelines for Americans, <www.health.gov/paguidelines>.

14. F Booth, et al (2012), "Lack of exercise is a major cause of chronic disease," *Comprehensive Physiology*, Vol 2, pages 1143-1211.

15. C W Hambrecht, et al (2004), "Percutaneous Coronary Angioplasty Compared With Exercise Training in Patients With Stable Coronary Artery Disease : A Randomized Trial," *Circulation*, Vol 109, pages 1371-8.

16. L S Pescatello, et al (2004), "Exercise and hypertension," *Medicine and Science in Sport and Exercise*, Vol 36 No 3, pages 533-53.

17. D Morton, et al (2013), "The effectiveness of the Complete Health Improvement Program (CHIP) in Australasia for reducing selected chronic disease risk factors: a feasibility study," *New Zealand Medical Journal*, Vol 126 No 1370, pages 43-54; P Rankin, et al (2012), "Effectiveness of a Volunteer-Delivered Lifestyle Modification Program for Reducing Cardiovascular Disease Risk Factors," *American Journal of Cardiology*, Vol 109, pages 82-6.

18. Rankin, op cit; see also P Rankin (2013),

"Effectiveness of the Complete Health Improvement Program (CHIP) lifestyle intervention for the management of the Metabolic Syndrome," Unpublished PhD dissertation.

19. R J Sigal (2006), "Physical Activity/Exercise and Type 2 Diabetes. A consensus statement from the American Diabetes Association," *Diabetes Care,* Vol 29 No 6, pages 1433-8.

20. M D Hordern, et al (2012), "Exercise prescription for patients with type 2 diabetes and pre-diabetes: A position statement from Exercise and Sport Science Australia," *Journal of Science and Medicine in Sport,* Vol 15 No 1, pages 25-31.

21. Baker IDI Heart and Diabetes Institute, "Lift for Life" <http://www.liftforlife.com.au/Page.aspx?ID=268>.

22. J Chavarro, et al (2007), "Diet and Lifestyle in the Prevention of Ovulatory Disorder Infertility," *Obstetrics & Gynecology,* Vol 110 No 5, pages 1050-8.

23. A Al-Mamari, et al (2009), "Atherosclerosis and physical activity," *Oman Medical Journal,* Vol 24, pages173-8.

24. H Mathur and B K Pedersen (2008), "Exercise as a Means to Control Low- Grade Systemic Inflammation," *Mediators of Inflammation,* Volume 2008, Article ID 109502.

25. ibid.

26. H Naci and J Ioannidis (2013), "Comparative effectiveness of exercise and drug interventions on mortality outcomes: metaepidemiological study," *British Journal of Medicine,* Vol 347, f5577.

27. U Schwarz, et al (2010), "Employee self rated productivity and objective organizational production levels," *Journal of Occupational and Environmental Medicine,* Vol 53 No 8, pages 838-44.

28. C Ernst, et al (2006), "Antidepressant effects of exercise: evidence for an adult-neurogenesis hypothesis?" *Journal of Psychiatry and Neuroscience,* Vol 31 No 2, pages 84-92.

29. A Strohle (2009), "Physical activity, exercise, depression and anxiety disorders," *Journal of Neural Transmission,* Vol 116, pages 777-84.

30. A F Kraemer and K I Erickson (2007), "Capitalizing on cortical plasticity: influence of PA on cognition and gut function," *Trends in Cognitive Science,* Vol 11 No 8, pages 342-8.

31. C W Cotman, et al (2007), "Exercise builds brain health: key roles of growth factor cascades and inflammation," *Trends in Neuroscience,* Vol 30 No 9, pages 464-71.

32. J Rosker and N Sarabon (2010), "Kinaesthesia and methods for its assessment," *Sports Science Reviews,* Vol XIX, No 5-6, pages 165-208.

33. Clark, op cit.

34. R Dishman and P O'Connor (2009), "Lessons in exercise neurobiology: the case for endorphins," *Mental Health and Physical Activity,* Vol 2, pages 4-9.

35. H Boecker (2008), "The runner's high: opioidergic mechanisms in the human brain," *Cerebral Cortex,* Vol 18 No 11, pages 1-9.

36. R Sapolsky (2004), *Why Zebras Don't Get Ulcers* (3rd edition), Henry Holt and Company.

37. J Opdenacker, et al (2009), "The longitudinal effects of a lifestyle physical activity intervention and a structured exercise intervention on physical self-perceptions and self-esteem in older adults," *Journal of Sport & Exercise Psychology,* Vol 31 No 6, pages 743-60.

38. L S Olive, et al. (2012), "Effect of physical activity, fitness and fatness on children's body image: the Australian LOOK longitudinal study," *Mental Health and Physical Activity,* Vol 5, pages 116-24.

39. World Health Organization (2012), <www.who.int/ mediacentre/factsheets/fs311/en/>.

40. G Danaei, et al (2009), "The preventable causes of death in the United States: comparative risk assessment of dietary, lifestyle, and metabolic risk factors," *PLOS online,* Vol 6, No 4, e1000058.

41. J Cloud (2010), "Why your DNA isn't your destiny," *Time,* January 6, 2010, <www.time.com/time/magazine/article/0,9171,19522313,00.html#ixzz24POuVP6g>.

42. I Janssen, et al (2004), "Waist circumference and not body mass index explains obesity-related health risk," *American Journal of Clinical Nutrition,* Vol 79, pages 379-84; S Zhu, et al (2002), "Waist circumference and obesity-associated risk factors among whites in the third National Health and Nutrition Examination Survey: clinical action thresholds," *American Journal of Clinical Nutrition,* Vol 76, pages 743-9.

43. J E Donnelly, et al (2009), "Appropriate Physical Activity Intervention Strategies for Weight Loss and Prevention of Weight Regain for Adults: American College of Sports Medicine Position Stand," *Medicine and Science in Sports and Exercise,* Special Communications, pages 459-71.

44. World Cancer Research Fund (2007), "Food, Nutrition, Physical Activity, and the prevention of cancer: a global perspective," *American Institute of Cancer Research.*

45. ibid.

46. Boecker, op cit.

47. C Martins, et al (2008), "A review of the effects of exercise on appetite regulation: an obesity perspective," *International Journal of Obesity,* Vol 32, pages 1337-47.

48. C Martins, et al (2010), "The Effects of Exercise-Induced Weight Loss on Appetite- Related Peptides and Motivation to Eat," *Journal of Clinical Endocrinology and Metabolism,* Vol 95 No 4, pages 1609-16.

49. R R Wing and S Phelan (2005), "Long-term weight loss maintenance," *American Journal of Clinical Nutrition,* Vol 82 No 1, pages 222S-5S; see also <www.nwcr.ws>.

50. J E Donnelly, op cit.

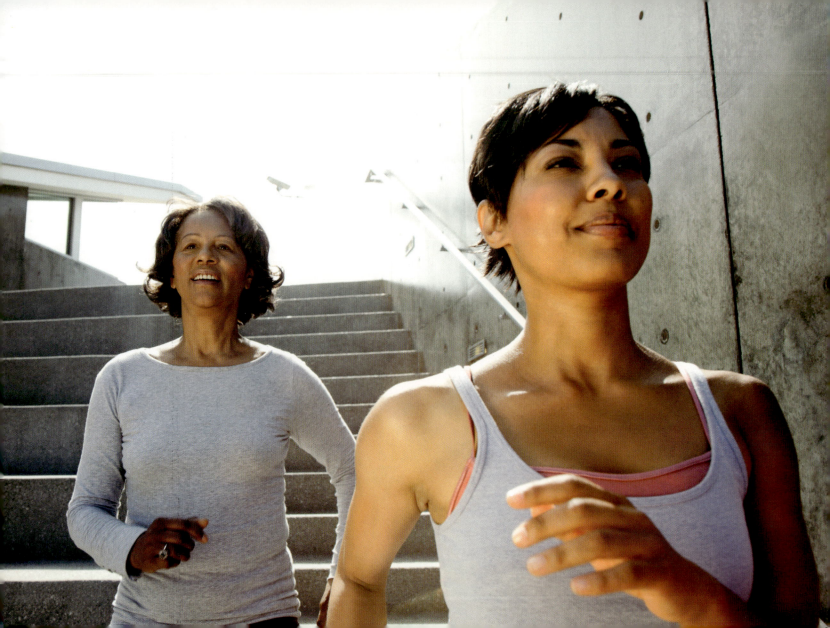

Chapter Four

Step 2: Oxygenate

In Step 1, you were encouraged to sit less and move more. And to help you keep track of how much you were moving throughout the day, you were introduced to the pedometer. But while counting steps can be a great way to monitor your daily physical activity—as you have probably already discovered—pedometers have limitations:

1. Pedometers don't count any of the steps you take if you forget to wear them.

2. There are many excellent forms of physical activity that pedometers don't count, such as swimming, cycling and resistance exercises (such as weightlifting).

3. Pedometers don't differentiate between the *type* of steps you take. Baby steps get counted no differently to "run-like-you-stole-something" steps. Hence, pedometers do not take into consideration the intensity of effort associated with the steps they count. As such, it is possible to achieve 10,000 steps without significantly increasing your breathing or heart rate, even though there are tremendous benefits for doing so.

For best health outcomes, you need to *oxygenate*, which brings us to Step 2 of the optimal active lifestyle.

> "I swam for 20 minutes, cycled for an hour and jogged for 20 minutes—it's been a big year!"

OXYGENATE

Oxygen is the most important nutrient required by your body for health, healing and life. You can survive for several weeks without food (it is not much fun—but you can), several days without water, but only a few minutes without oxygen.

There is no better way to deliver oxygen to your body than through "aerobic" physical activity. *Aerobic* simply means "with oxygen"—and aerobic activities are those physical pursuits that cause an increase in breathing and heart rates. As such, aerobic activities improve the *fitness* of your cardio-respiratory system, which in turn helps protect against diseases of the heart, lungs and blood vessels that constitute the biggest killers in developed countries.

SLOWING THE BEAT

As you improve your aerobic fitness, it is not uncommon for your resting heart rate to decrease—sometimes by as much as 10 beats per minute in the first 10 weeks of exercising. This occurs because the heart becomes stronger and can pump more blood with each beat and therefore doesn't have to beat as often. Elite athletes have been known to have a resting heart rate of less than 30 beats per minute, less than half the rate of an average adult (typically 70-80 beats per minute).

Research has demonstrated that aerobic exercise confers these health benefits independent of weight loss. Obese individuals who are active have lower morbidity and mortality rates than normal-weight but sedentary individuals.[1] This shows that being fit will ameliorate many of the health hazards of being obese,[2] which highlights that exercise does great things on the inside, even if not noticeable from the outside. Perhaps we should be more concerned with fitness than fatness.

30 MINUTES, MOST DAYS

Aerobic exercise was first popularized more than 40 years ago by Dr Kenneth Cooper, who began to research its effect on health and wellbeing.[3] Dr Cooper's research grew into the world-leading Aerobic Center Longitudinal Study, which now involves more than 250,000 records from around 100,000 individuals.[4] One of the key findings of this study is that individuals who participate in around 150 minutes of moderate-intensity aerobic exercise

THE RISK OF DYING PREMATURELY DECLINES AS PEOPLE ENGAGE IN MORE AEROBIC EXERCISE

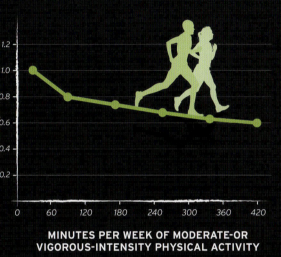

MINUTES PER WEEK OF MODERATE-OR VIGOROUS-INTENSITY PHYSICAL ACTIVITY

The Aerobic Center Longitudinal Study has shown that individuals who participate in around 150 minutes of moderate-intensity aerobic exercise each week—about 30 minutes most days—have a greatly reduced risk of premature death.

Examples of EXERCISE

Moderate-intensity physical activity includes:
- GENTLE SWIMMING
- SOCIAL TENNIS
- PURPOSEFUL WALKING
- GENTLE CYCLING

Vigorous-intensity physical activity includes:
- JOGGING
- CYCLING FAST
- AEROBIC CLASSES
- COMPETITIVE TENNIS

each week—about 30 minutes most days—have a greatly reduced risk of premature death.

Recognizing this finding, many countries have developed physical activity guidelines that include the goal of "30 minutes of moderate-intensity physical activity most days" as a recommendation for adults, including older adults, and twice this amount for children.[5] Further research has indicated that the 30 minutes can be broken down into three 10-minute blocks that can be spread throughout the day, which is hardly surprising given that we don't eat our daily supply of food for the day in the one sitting. This is good news for individuals who struggle to find a free 30-minute chunk in their day.

Now if you are thinking, "Oh, no! Here is where it gets hard!"—relax. While there are additional benefits gained from engaging in "vigorous-intensity" aerobic activity, the bulk of the benefits come from engaging in only "moderate-intensity" aerobic activity. Contrary to the popular saying, there can be great gain with no pain!

So what's the difference between moderate-intensity and vigorous-intensity physical activity?

Moderate-intensity exercise causes a noticeable increase in breathing rate but you can still maintain an uninterrupted conversation. Such an intensity could be maintained for 30 to 60 minutes and would rate as an effort of 3- or 4-out-of-10.[6] Examples of moderate-intensity physical activity might include: gentle swimming, social tennis, walking with a purpose, or cycling at a regular pace.

Vigorous-intensity exercise describes physical activities during which a conversation could not be maintained uninterrupted—you would need to catch your breath between sentences. The intensity could usually not be sustained for more than 30 minutes at a time and it would rate as a 5- or 6-out-of-10 effort.[7] Vigorous-intensity physical activity might include jogging, cycling fast, aerobic classes, and competitive tennis.

....

Note: Intensity of effort is a personal thing, relative to your fitness level. One individual's "moderate-intensity" might be a slow walk, while for someone else it might be a jog.

....

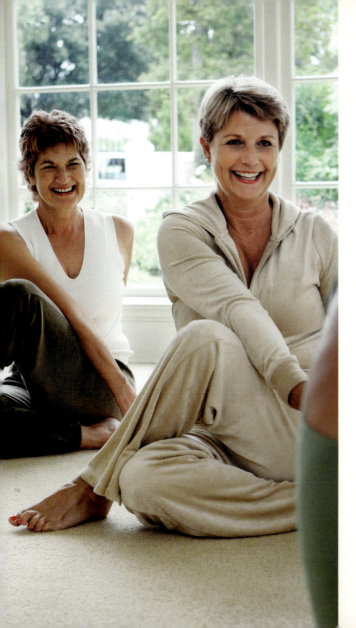

DAY 9

GET WITH THE BEAT

Another popular way of judging how taxing a certain exercise level is on your body is to monitor your heart rate. Personally, I like to keep it simple. Unless you are training for high-level fitness, subjectively gauging your level of intensity—self-rating how hard you are finding it and taking note of how much you are breathing—is sufficient. That said, some people find monitoring their heart rate interesting and helpful. Certainly, measuring heart rate can provide a more accurate objective measure of how intensely your body is working during exercise, although it should be noted that your heart rate can fluctuate from day to day. Factors such as dehydration can also cause your heart rate to be higher for the same exercise intensity.

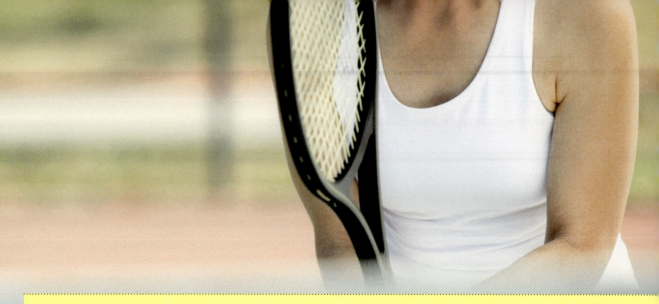
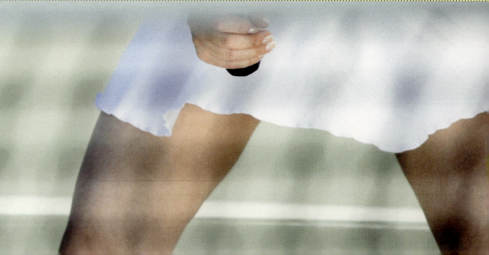

CLASSIFYING THE INTENSITY OF EXERCISE[8]

The table shows how heart rate can be used to determine how intensely you are exercising. For more information about how to calculate your "heart rate," see Section 2.

Intensity category	Objective measure	Subjective measure	Descriptive measure
Sedentary	<40% maximum heart rate	< 1 out of 10 in effort	Activities that usually involve sitting or lying and that have little additional movement and a low energy requirement.
Light	40-55% maximum heart rate	1-2 out of 10 in effort	An aerobic activity that does not cause a noticeable change in breathing rate. An intensity that can be sustained for at least 60 minutes.
Moderate	55-70% maximum heart rate	3-4 out of 10 in effort	An aerobic activity that is able to be conducted while maintaining an uninterrupted conversation. An intensity that can be sustained between 30-60 minutes.
Vigorous	70-90% maximum heart rate	5-6 out of 10 in effort	An aerobic activity in which a conversation generally cannot be maintained uninterrupted. An intensity that generally cannot be sustained for longer than about 30 minutes.
High	>90% maximum heart rate	>7 out of 10 in effort	An intensity that generally cannot be sustained for longer than about 10 minutes.

DAY 10

THE EXTRA BENEFITS OF GOING VIGOROUS

Have you ever noticed after exercise you feel warm for some time later—a type of "after-burn"? That after-burn feeling typically persists for two hours after the exercise session, but it can continue for up to 48 hours,[9] during which time you can burn another 15 per cent of the energy used during the exercise that started it.[10]

For many years—and sometimes still today—individuals were instructed to go "low (intensity) and slow" to lose body fat. This was based on the observation that during low-intensity exercise the body tends to utilize fat for energy, whereas during higher intensity activities it relies more on carbohydrate.[11] But the source of energy that the body uses during exercise is less important than the total amount of energy used. Higher intensities are better in this regard.

It is not surprising that there is an emerging body of evidence showing that more vigorous-intensity activities achieve better weight loss than lower intensities.[12] For example, in a study of women who either cycled at a constant moderate-intensity or performed repeated bouts of eight seconds fast followed by 12 seconds slow, the women who performed the short bursts of intensity experienced significantly greater decreases in body fat from their legs and trunk.[13]

EXERCISE ON AN EMPTY STOMACH FOR FAT LOSS?

A common fat-burning strategy is to exercise early in the morning on an empty stomach. The rationale is that, in a fasted state, your body is forced to rely more on stored fat for energy.

There is no good evidence to support this idea. In fact, when you exercise after eating, a greater amount of energy is used to digest the meal.[14] Obviously, there are limits to this—exercising on a full stomach can cause gastrointestinal upset.

The take-away message: Eating before or after exercise is neither here nor there, the most important thing is you exercise!

Another benefit of vigorous-intensity over moderate-intensity exercise is that it can be twice as time-efficient. Because vigorous-intensity exercise oxygenates your body more effectively than moderate-intensity activity, you don't have to do as much of it to achieve the same outcomes. To get the same benefits as 30 minutes of moderate-intensity activity, you probably only need to perform 15 minutes of vigorous-intensity exercise—essentially you can apply a 2-to-1 ratio.[15] For this reason, the United States and Australian physical activity guidelines state that adults should aim for 150 minutes of moderate-intensity physical activity each week (30 minutes, five days a week) or only 75 minutes of vigorous-intensity physical activity. For those who are time-pressed, this makes vigorous-intensity exercise more attractive.

In a study of more than 1400 men diagnosed with early-stage prostate cancer, those who walked briskly for at least three hours a week were 57 per cent less likely to have their cancer progress than those who walked less often and less vigorously. In another study, men diagnosed with localized prostate cancer who engaged in vigorous activity at least three hours each week had a 61 per cent lower chance of dying from the illness, compared to men who engaged in vigorous activity less than one hour a week.[16]

TAKE A H-I-T

There is currently great interest in a form of exercise referred to as HIT (High-intensity Interval Training) that shows promise as an extremely time-efficient method for achieving exercise-induced health benefits.[17] HIT involves short bursts of high-intensity exercise for brief periods (10-30 seconds) followed by long rest periods (1 to 4 minutes). One study found that healthy but sedentary individuals who performed 10 minutes of HIT involving only two high-intensity bursts interspersed with low-intensity recovery improved their insulin sensitivity by nearly 30 per cent after only six weeks.[18] Indeed, it seems that exercise intensity is more important than exercise duration for improving insulin sensitivity, which is especially significant for people with diabetes.[19]

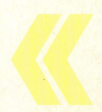

Caution: Because vigorous-intensity exercise circulates oxygen and other nutrients to your body more dynamically, it presents a greater challenge to your heart muscle. This is a good thing if you are used to it—it makes your heart stronger—but if you are not accustomed to it, you should work up to it slowly and get medical clearance if you answer "yes" to any of the questions in the Physical Activity Readiness Questionnaire below. For those accustomed to vigorous exercise, it is estimated that the chance of having a heart attack during vigorous-intensity exercise is one in 1.57 million.[20]

PHYSICAL ACTIVITY READINESS QUESTIONNAIRE

> If you answer "yes" to one or more questions, are older than age 40 and have been inactive, or are concerned about your health, it is a good idea to get a checkup with your doctor before getting "vigorous."

1. Has your doctor ever said that you have a heart condition and that you should only do physical activity recommended by a doctor?

2. Do you feel pain in your chest when you do physical activity?

3. In the past month, have you had chest pain when you were not doing physical activity?

4. Do you lose your balance because of dizziness or do you ever lose consciousness?

5. Do you have a bone or joint problem that could be made worse by a change in your physical activity?

6. Is your doctor currently prescribing medication for your blood pressure or heart condition?

7. Do you know of any other reason why you should not do physical activity?

A final added benefit of performing vigorous-intensity exercise is that it makes you feel more vigorous. I find that when I only perform low-intensity exercise, I don't have as much spring in my step as when I intentionally include elements of more vigorous-intensity exercise. Who doesn't want that spring!

However, while engaging in vigorous-intensity exercise does confer extra benefits, I must stress that the bulk of the benefits come from performing moderate-intensity activity, so don't feel compelled to go harder. If you are willing and able to include elements of vigorous-intensity exercise into your routine, start by interspersing short periods of higher-intensity exercise (10 seconds or so at first) and build up as your fitness improves.

HOW IS AEROBIC FITNESS MEASURED?

The gold standard for measuring an individual's aerobic fitness is the Maximal Oxygen Uptake (VO_2max) test, typically performed on a treadmill or bicycle ergometer. The individual starts exercising at a low intensity, which is incrementally increased every minute or so while the air they expire is analysed to determine how much oxygen they are using. The maximal amount of oxygen the individual consumes as they reach exhaustion is deemed their VO_2max. The maximal oxygen uptake of an average male is around 35-40 ml/kg/min but highly trained elite athletes can have a value more than twice this amount—five-time Tour de France winner Miguel Indurain was reported to have a VO_2max of 88 ml/kg/min, which is huge. Women's' average scores are closer to 30 ml/kg/min. As the body uses the oxygen to generate energy, an individual with a higher VO_2max clearly has an advantage in sports and activities that make you puff.

DAY 11

MORE IS BETTER FOR STAYING SLIM

The current guidelines for most developed countries recommend 30 minutes of moderate-intensity aerobic activity most days. This is a worthwhile goal—especially given that three out of four adults in the United States don't achieve it.[21] But there is growing evidence urging that more is better.

Without wanting to be discouraging or overwhelming, several studies now suggest that, because we have become so sedentary, 30 minutes of moderate-intensity physical activity a day may not be enough, particularly for controlling body weight. One expert panel has suggested that formerly obese individuals who want to keep the weight off may need to perform as much as 60 to 90 minutes of moderate-intensity physical activity a day.[22]

This recommendation is in line with the findings of the National Weight Control Registry, which has reported that individuals who successfully lose a significant portion of weight and keep it off consistently engage in about one hour of moderate-intensity physical activity every day.[23] The position of the American College of Sports Medicine states that it is ideal to aim for 250-300 minutes per week of moderate-intensity physical activity,[24] which works out to be 50-60 minutes, five days a week. The recent Australian Physical Activity and Sedentary Behaviour Guidelines concur.[26] If this amount of activity seems excessive, it is only because we have become so accustomed to sedentary living. We have come to think of sitting around and not moving as "normal"—but this is not the way our bodies see it. Remember, we are made to move!

CAN YOU BE TOO ACTIVE?

You can get too much of a good thing, including exercise. Athletes who exercise too much with inadequate recovery can develop a condition referred to as the "overtraining syndrome." Athletes experiencing overtraining syndrome are more susceptible to flus and other viruses, experience fatigue and performance decline, and suffer mood disturbances.[25]

So how much is too much? The answer is different from person to person as we all have different capacities, but if you follow the principles of the optimal active lifestyle outlined in this book, this is not something you need to worry about.

Chapter Four References

1. S N Blair and S Brodney (1999), "Effects of physical inactivity and obesity on morbidity and mortality: current evidence and research issues," *Medicine and Science in Sports and Exercise*, Vol 31 No 11 Supplement, pages S646-62.

2. D C Lee, et al (2009), "Does physical activity ameliorate the health hazards of obesity?" *British Journal of Sports Medicine*, Vol 43, pages 49-51; D C Lee, et al (2011), "Long- Term Effects of Changes in Cardiorespiratory Fitness and Body Mass Index on All-Cause and Cardiovascular Disease Mortality in Men: The Aerobics Center Longitudinal Study," *Circulation*, Vol 124, pages 2483-90.

3. K Cooper (1969), *Aerobics*, Bantam Books.

4. <www.cooperaerobics.com>.

5. United States Department of Health and Human Services, "2008 Physical Activity Guidelines for Americans," <www.health.gov/paguidelines>; see also Active Australia (1999), "Physical Activity Guidelines for Adults," <http://www.healthyactive.gov.au>.

6. K Norton, et al (2010), "Position statement on physical activity and exercise intensity terminology," *Journal of Science and Medicine in Sport*, Vol 13, pages 496-502.

7. ibid.

8. Adapted from Norton, ibid.

9. J Laforgia, et al (2006), "Effects of exercise intensity and duration on the excess post-exercise oxygen consumption," *Journal of Sports Sciences*, Vol 24 No 12, pages 1247-64;
C A Vella, et al (2006), "Exercise After-Burn: A Research Update," *IDEA Fitness Journal*, Vol 1 No 4, <www.ideafit.com/fitness-library/exercise-after-burn-0>.

10. J R Speakman, et al (2003), "Physical activity and resting metabolic rate," *Proceedings of the Nutrition Society*, Vol 62, pages 621-34.

11. W D McArdle, et al (2009), *Exercise Physiology: Nutrition, energy and human performance*, Lippincott Williams & Wilkins.

12. B Schonenfeld, et al (2009), "High-Intensity Interval Training: Applications for General Fitness Training," *Strength and Conditioning Journal*, Vol 31 No 6, pages 44-6.

13. E G Trapp, et al (2008), "The effects of high-intensity intermittent exercise training on fat loss and fasting insulin levels of young women," *International Journal of Obesity*, Vol 32 No 4, pages 684-91.

14. B Schonenfeld (2011), "Does Cardio After an Overnight Fast Maximize Fat Loss?" *Strength and Conditioning Journal*, Vol 33 No 1, pages 23-5.

15. United States Department of Health and Human Services, "2008 Physical Activity Guidelines for Americans," <www.health.gov/paguidelines>; World Health Organization (2010), "Global recommendations on physical activity for health," <whqlibdoc.who.int/publications/2010/9789241599979_eng.pdf>.

16. Harvard Medical School (2013), "Annual Report on Prostate Diseases," Harvard Health Publications.

17. M J Gibala, et al (2012), "Physiological adaptations to low-volume, high-intensity interval training in health and disease," *Journal of Physiology*, Vol 590 No 5, pages 1077-84; H S Kessler, et al (2012), "The Potential for High-Intensity Interval Training to Reduce Cardiometabolic Disease Risk," *Sports Medicine*, Vol 42 No 6, pages 489-509.

18. R S Metcalfe, et al (2012), "Towards the minimal amount of exercise for improving metabolic health: beneficial effects of reduced-exertion high-intensity interval training," *European Journal of Applied Physiology*, Vol 112 No 7, pages 2767-75.

19. M D Hordern, et al (2012), "Exercise prescription for patients with type 2 diabetes and pre-diabetes: A position statement from Exercise and Sport Science Australia," *Journal of Science and Medicine in Sport*, Vol 15, pages 25-31.

20. J Erlichman, et al (2012), "Physical activity and its impact on health outcomes. Paper 1: the impact of physical activity on cardiovascular disease and all-cause mortality: an historical perspective," *Obesity Reviews*, Vol 3, pages 257-71.

21. R Brownson, et al (2005), "Declining rates of physical activity in the United States: what are the contributors?" *American Review of Public Health*, Vol 26, pages 421-43.

22. W H Saris, et al (2003), "How much physical activity is enough to prevent unhealthy weight gain? Outcome of the IASO 1st Stock Conference and consensus statement," *Obesity Reviews*, Vol 4, pages 101-14.

23. National Weight Control Registry, <www.nwcr.ws>.

24. J E Donnelly, et al (2009), "Appropriate Physical Activity Intervention Strategies for Weight Loss and Prevention of Weight Regain for Adults: American College of Sports Medicine Position Stand," *Medicine and Science in Sports and Exercise*, Special Communications, pages 459-71.

25. R Meeusen, et al (2006), "Prevention, diagnosis and treatment of the Overtraining Syndrome," *European Journal of Sport Science*, Vol 6 No 1, pages 1-14.

26. Department of Health (2014), "Australia's Physical Activity and Sedentary Behaviour Guidelines," <www.health.gov.au/internet/main/publishing.nsf/content/health-pubhlth-strateg-phys-act-guidelines>.

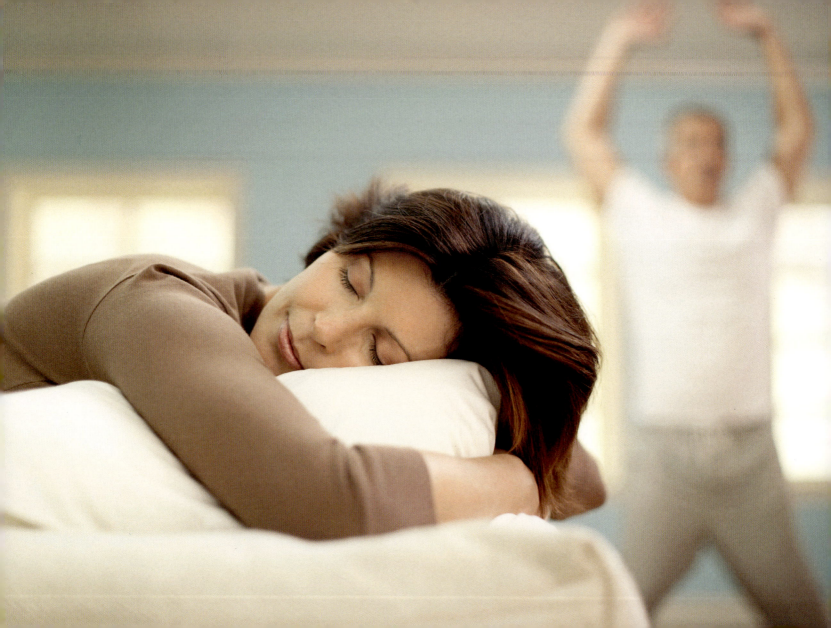

DAY 12

Chapter Five

Excuses, excuses!

"If it is important to you, you will find a way. If it is not, you will find an excuse."

When it comes to excuses for not being active, I have heard them all:

> "The boss dumped a huge pile of work on my desk."
>
> "I started to come down with a sore throat and thought it best to rest."
>
> "I wasn't sure how to do the exercise right and figured I was better to be safe than sorry."

Of course, our excuses usually involve extenuating circumstances for explaining why we didn't do what we know we should have. Less often do we cite the real reasons for our inactivity such as:

> "I couldn't be bothered."
>
> "It is so boring."
>
> "I don't like it."

At some times on your journey toward the optimal active lifestyle, you are going to feel the urge to excuse why you don't need to be active today. Before these excuses become showstoppers, let's deal with them upfront. Of course, I'm not suggesting there is never a legitimate excuse for not moving much, but if you are honest, you will agree that we excuse ourselves more often than we ought.

So let's examine 10 common excuses people use for avoiding exercise. In essence, they represent the common barriers people face to being physically active. Some of them are legitimate concerns and the responses below will help alleviate them—or at least provide ideas for best negotiating them. Other excuses listed below are simply those we use to justify our lack of enthusiasm and make ourselves feel better about it. The responses to these excuses might be just what you need to hear in order to prevent them getting in your way.

1. I don't have the time to exercise.

Lack of time is often reported as the major barrier to being active.[1] While it is true that the pace of life today seems faster than ever, let's be honest. Do you find time to watch TV or surf the internet? Do you find the time to eat regularly? The truth is time is not the problem for most people; the problem is prioritizing.

Steven Covey—author of *The 7 Habits of Highly Effective People* and *First Things First*—has an excellent analogy for representing how we prioritize our time. He starts with an empty bucket, which represents the time we have available to us in a day.

He then places some big rocks in the bucket that represent the truly important things we should put in our day like time with family and friends, time for personal growth and time for physical activity.

He then poses the question, "Is the bucket full?" Of course, it isn't. There are spaces between the big rocks, so he fills these spaces with smaller rocks that represent the lesser important but nonetheless necessary things we must get into our day—work, meetings, dropping the kids off at soccer practice.

He then asks the question again: "Is the bucket full?" Clearly there are still gaps between the smaller rocks. By shaking the bucket and moving it around he manages to fill even the smallest cracks with sand, representing the many unimportant time-wasters that often jam-pack our days.

At the end of the demonstration, he poses the question, "What is the point of the analogy?" It is tempting to think the take-away message is to shuffle our timetable so we can pack in more and more to our day. But this is not the lesson. Instead, Covey explains that if we don't put the big rocks in first, we will never get them in. [2]

Time for physical activity needs to be one of the big rocks placed in your bucket first. Deciding before the day starts when you will be active greatly increases the likelihood that you will do it, so plan ahead.

If your lack of time can't be resolved by better prioritizing the truly important things in life—relationships and positive health behaviors such as physical activity—you are too busy and something needs to change. If you don't *choose* to make changes, you will likely be *forced* to by the consequences of your poor lifestyle practices. We all have hectic periods in life—but living a frantic pace is not sustainable in the long-term.

In the pursuit of living more, taking time for regular physical activity is a non-negotiable. Besides, it need not be time intensive—just capturing 10-minute chunks throughout the day works wonders, as we have seen.

2. Exercise is too dangerous!

We have all heard stories—perhaps from a friend of a friend of a friend—of the person who went jogging and suddenly dropped dead. Just goes to show: exercise is far too dangerous! What is told less often is how infrequently this happens.

Among the general population, the chance of sudden death during exercise from a heart attack is estimated to be between 0 to 2 episodes per 100,000 exercise hours. And among those with a known heart condition participating in a cardiac rehabilitation program, estimates are from 0.13 to 0.61 episodes per 100,000 exercise hours.[3]

For most people, there is no reason why they should be fearful about increasing their physical activity levels.[4] However, as previously discussed, it's a good idea to get a checkup from your doctor before engaging in vigorous activities if you are not accustomed to it, just for peace of mind. Of course, it is also wise to listen to your body. If you notice signs that things are not well—especially pain in your chest, left arm or neck—slow down and follow it up immediately.

Finally, even if exercise is risky—which statistics show it isn't—the alternative is lethal. For every person who perishes while perspiring, millions die prematurely with a poor quality of life because they are underactive. In fact, if I have enough vitality to be jogging on the day I die, I'll be delighted. It is better than the fate of many inactive individuals who can expect years of illness leading up to their death.

So it is a good idea to get the all-clear from your doctor before getting serious with an exercise program, but don't let the thought that exercise is dangerous stop you—the benefits clearly outweigh the risks.

3. I am sick, injured or health problems prevent me from being active.

If you are at death's door, you are justified in lying down and concentrating only on breathing—but people often use mild sickness or injury as an excuse to do nothing.

For example, a sore leg does not mean you need to immobilize your arms. I once had an injury to my right thigh that persisted for six weeks. My solution was to take the right pedal off my bike and ride furiously with my left leg. I attracted some stares from passers-by—but it worked a treat.

There is usually something we can find to do if we are creative. If one body part is injured, activate another part that isn't. The same applies if you have a more permanent health condition that restricts your ability to be active. Just do what you can. Remember, everything helps.

Story: When John Maclean lost the use of his legs, it didn't slow him down—if anything he sped up! Although clearly devastated in the wake of the accident that left him a paraplegic, John went on to complete the Hawaiian Ironman triathlon, which involves a 2.4-mile (3.8-kilometer) swim, 110-mile (180-kilometer) cycle and 26-mile (42-kilometer) run—just the run is a full marathon. Contesting the event in his modified, arm-cranked bicycle and "racing chair," John was the first para-athlete to make the able-bodied cut-off time for the event. As if that is not enough, John has also swum the English Channel. Inspirational stories like John's can help put things in perspective.[5]

When it comes to more systemic illnesses like the flu, a good policy is to apply the "neck check."[6] If your symptoms are confined to above your neck, such as a head cold or sore throat, it is probably OK to engage in light activity. Go for a casual stroll. However, if the symptoms present below the neck-line, such as a chesty cough and achy body, it is best to rest entirely.

DAY 13

> ### Does exercise boost your immune system?
>
> The immune system is extremely complex, but several studies have examined the influence of exercise on upper respiratory tract infections. The relationship between the incidence of upper respiratory tract infections and the amount of exercise we perform can be described by a "J" curve—moderately active individuals have a 20 to 30 per cent lower risk of contracting a cold than sedentary people, but extreme exercisers are at the greatest risk.[7] Other infectious diseases may follow a similar pattern.
>
> This suggests that moderate amounts of exercise boosts the immune system but excessive exercise, as performed by some athletes, may suppress it. Importantly, with the level of activity represented by the optimal active lifestyle, you can expect a boost to your immunity!

4. I have too many stressful things going on to exercise.

At times, life throws stressful events at us that can derail our resolve and it is one of the most common obstacles to more active living. Yet even in our most stressful periods, it is a good idea to prioritize being physically active as it can help keep us sane. I have a friend who is the principal of a large high school with no shortage of challenges and stresses. He claims that as his stress levels increase, so too does the length of his daily walk.

As discussed in Chapter 3, physical activity is one of the best things we can do to manage stress and so the busier and more stressful life becomes for you, the more important it is that you keep physically active—it can be your lifeline.

5. The weather is no good.

There is no doubt that you feel more like being active outdoors when the weather is agreeable, and less inclined when the weather is miserable. But there are plenty of indoor activity options, so "bad" weather is not a legitimate excuse.

That said, I recommend exercising outdoors whenever you can, especially in natural environments.

So many people today spend the bulk of their time indoors, alienated from the natural world that we are designed to inhabit. In fact, a new term has been coined: Nature Deficit Disorder (NDD). Children suffering Nature Deficit Disorder—those who don't get to regularly spend time outdoors—are more prone to anxiety, depression, attention deficit disorder and even being overweight.[8] Outdoors we can find fresh air and sunlight, both of which can do us much good.

Clearly there are limits to the environmental extremes in which we should be active. Hot and humid conditions can be potentially dangerous and it is best to exercise early in the morning or later in the evening in these climates. Similarly, extreme cold can be hazardous and appropriate care should be taken—although I have a doctor friend from Canada where -4F (-20C) is not uncommon during winter who says, "There is no bad weather, just bad clothing."

Given the many alternatives, "bad" weather doesn't really cut it as an excuse for not moving.

6. I don't know what to do.

The notion of exercising for the sake of exercising is a relatively new thing for the general population. Going back only a century or so, we didn't need to be intentional about moving our bodies because our daily living demanded it. It is only because our days are commonly filled with inactivity that we need to be purposeful about taking time to exercise. Remember, we are designed to be active and things go wrong if we aren't.

Unfortunately, the concept of "exercise" has been made so complicated and it is little wonder that people are puzzled about what to do. We are bombarded by information about the latest exercise that you only have to do for "three minutes a week to achieve rock-hard tummy muscles" or specialized zones in which you need to set your heart rate to burn fat. But it shouldn't be confusing, and you will find everything you need to know regarding what to do in this book. Be sure to engage with Section 2. This excuse won't stop you now!

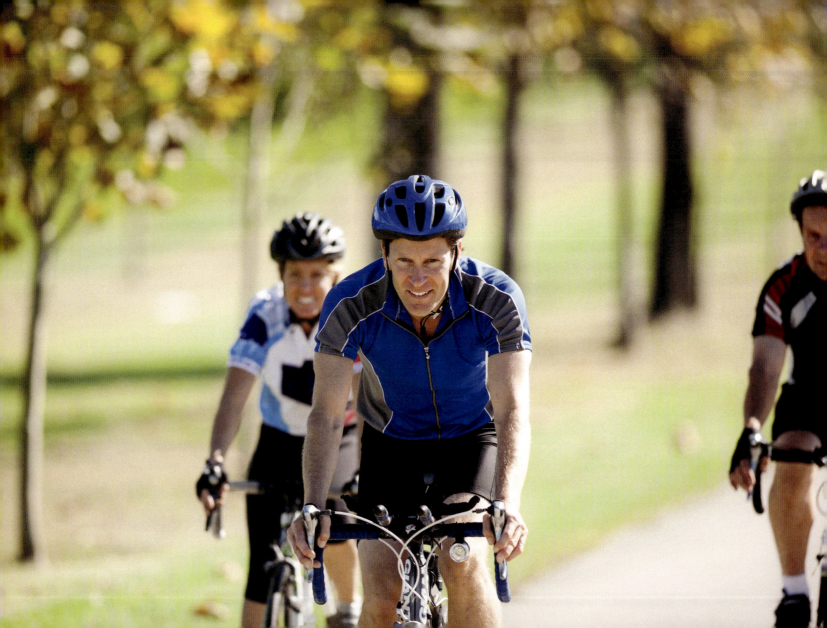

7. Exercise is boring and I don't like it!

If you find yourself using this excuse out loud, thank you for being honest. But to put it in perspective, I don't look forward to brushing my teeth but I do it because I recognize its benefits—for both myself and others! There are many things in life that don't fill us with joy but we still do them because they are important.

However, it is important to make your exercise time as enjoyable as possible. To achieve this, find something you do enjoy doing. There are so many options available so experiment with various movement opportunities until you find something you don't detest. Having more than one exercise option is another good way to relieve boredom—I alternate between swimming, running, cycling, paddling and doing resistance exercises so I never get bored.

Try also adding other stimulating elements to your exercise time—listen to music or an audiobook, exercise in different locations, or do it with others. Finally, don't push it too hard if that is not your style. While some people get a kick out of pushing themselves—and good on them if they do it safely—remember that exercise doesn't need to be unbearably painful.

Encouragingly, I know of many sworn exercise-haters who have come to thoroughly enjoy it in time. But it does take time, so persist through the early stages until those endorphins begin to turn exercise from a drag to a joy.

> **Story:** Social activist and filmmaker Michael Moore happened upon walking in a surreptitious way. After posting on his blog one Saturday night how depressing he found the statistic that more people in the United States are on antidepressant medications than go to the movies, someone suggested that walking might be the antidote. To test it out, Michael stepped outside and went walking. Several hundred nights later, he is still walking. And why? He comments, "I feel great. I can see my feet! There they are! Hello, feet! Wanna go for a walk? The feet say YES! Ask yours right now."[9]

8. I'm too tired, old or just can't be bothered.

Let's start with the "I'm-just-too-tired" excuse. There are times when the most important thing you can do for your quality of life is lie down and rest. But often those who claim they are too "exhausted" to exercise are the ones who drive to work, sit at their desk all day moving only their finger muscles on a keyboard, then drive home to collapse into the recliner. They should be bursting with energy because they have hardly expended any all day! Conversely, active people are usually the ones who seem to have energy to burn at the end of the day.

There is a profound irony that applies to most areas of our lives: "The more you give, the more you get." Certainly, this applies—within limits—to your energy levels. When you get into the habit of using energy, as occurs during exercise, your body expands its energy reserves. It does this according to the "overload principle"—when you extend your body beyond what it is accustomed to, it responds by adapting to cope and function better in the future. The overload principle explains why muscles get stronger in response to lifting weights and the heart gets more efficient in response to brisk walking.

With regard to being too old, you are never too old. At any age, being physically active (within your ability) is an essential ingredient for living more. In fact, national physical activity recommendations are the same for older adults as they are for younger adults.[10]

Finally, for those who just can't be bothered, my advice is two-fold.

First, go over the reasons why being physically active is so essential, as we have already seen, and be sure to engage with Section 2 in which you are guided through an exercise to help these reasons move you.

Next, just start *something*. Just put on your walking shoes and get out the front door. Once you are on a roll, it is easy to keep rolling. Simply moving in an energetic manner causes you to feel more energetic. I often tell people who can't be bothered going for a half-hour walk to just go for five minutes. I then add, "If after the five minutes you feel like it, go for another 25 minutes!" It is amazing how just five minutes of walking can evaporate the "I-can't-be-bothered" feeling.

9. I don't have the facilities or the money.

You don't need expensive equipment or a gym memberships to be active. There is plenty you can do with minimal equipment—you can be your own gym!

Throughout this book, I have intentionally presented exercises and activities that require minimal, easily accessible equipment so this excuse does not need to hinder you.

In addition, there are many free activity options that you can access. There is no charge for walking, and walking paths are provided in many places. Freely accessible outdoor exercise equipment is also becoming increasingly popular.

10. I feel embarrassed.

On one hand, I can understand that someone who is not in good shape might feel embarrassed to be seen exercising in front of others who are physically fit. People often comment that they don't like to go to gyms for this reason. But let me share a different perspective.

When I see someone who is carrying a bit of extra weight out exercising, my instant thought is, "What a legend!" I feel genuinely proud of them and want to cheer them on. And I am not alone in thinking this way. I have competed at a high level in triathlons and other events. On many occasions after finishing with the front-runners, I have stood with them at the finish line cheering on the rest of the field. And it is always those at the back of the pack who excite the greatest cheers. There is no condemnation, only praise.

So don't feel embarrassed. Feel proud! There are many onlookers applauding your efforts.

Now I recognize that there are mockers, but they don't rate a mention. Don't let them stop you—it is not about them, it's all about your journey and the wonders you are working for *you*. As Theodore Roosevelt said, "It's not the critic who counts. Credit belongs to the man (or woman) who is in the arena." I have a good friend who has—in her own words—gone from "fat to fit." She says that when she first started she would say to herself, "At least I am lapping everyone sitting on the sofa!"

DAY 14

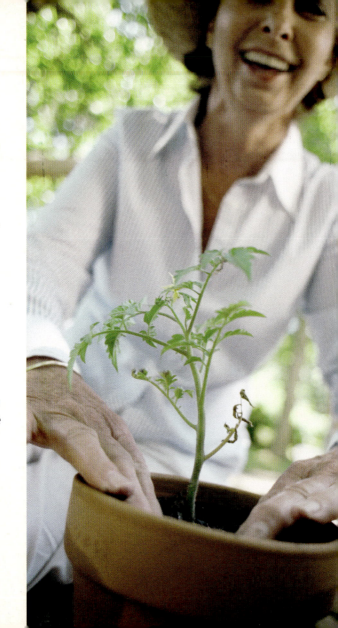

Overcoming the barriers

The more barriers you have to being active—even if they are just perceived—the less likely you are to follow through and be active.[11] In this section, we have addressed the most common barriers, which often masquerade as excuses, so they don't get in the way of you living more active. Be sure to re-read the appropriate sections if the excuses raise their head again. Dealing with our excuses is an important step toward making the transition to a more active lifestyle.

However, being excuse-free does not guarantee we will actually follow through and activate our life. In a large study that examined people's barriers to exercising, more than 40 per cent of those who claimed to not have any excuses for not being active still did not act! (See the graph on the following page.) More is required to be set for success on a behavior-change journey, as we shall explore as we progress toward the optimal active lifestyle.

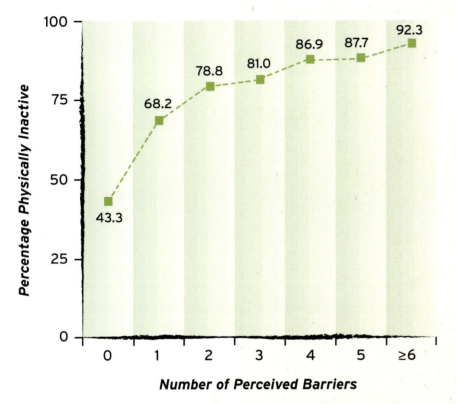

Prevalence of leisure-time physical inactivity and the number of perceived barriers to physical activity.[12]

Chapter Five References

1. F F Riechert, et al (2007), "The Role of Perceived Personal Barriers to Engagement in Leisure-Time Physical Activity," *American Journal of Public Health*, Vol 97 No 3, pages 515–9.

2. See S Covey (1996), *First Things First* (reprinted edition), Free Press, pages 88–9.

3. G F Fletcher, et al (1992), "Statement on exercise: Benefits and recommendations for physical activity programs for all Americans—A statement for health professionals by the Committee on Exercise and Cardiac Rehabilitation of the Council on Clinical Cardiology, American Heart Association," *Circulation*, Vol 86 No 1, pages 340–4.

4. L S Pescatello, et al (2004), "Exercise and Hypertension," *Medicine & Science in Sports & Exercise*, Vol 36 No 3, pages 533–53.

5. D Morton (2003), "Inspirational Tale: David Knight," *NETWORK for Fitness Professionals*, May edition, pages 18–19.

6. R Eichner (1995), "Contagious infections in competitive sports," *Sports Science Exchange*, Vol 8 No 3, <http://www.gssiweb.org/Article/sse-56-contagious-infections-in-competitive-sports>.

7. M Harris (2011), "Infectious diseases in athletes," *Current Sports Medicine Reports*, Vol 10 No 2, pages 84–9.

8. R Louv (2011), *The Nature Principle: Human Restoration and the End of Nature-Deficit Disorder*, Algonquin Books.

9. <http://www.facebook.com/mmflint/posts/10151165307981857>.

10. United States Department of Health and Human Services, "2008 Physical Activity Guidelines for Americans," <www.health.gov/paguidelines>.

11. Reichert, op cit.

12. ibid.

DAY 15

Chapter Six

Step 3: Strengthen and Stretch

> Congratulations on making it to Step 3—the final step toward the optimal active lifestyle! Step 1 simply involved sitting less and moving more throughout the day. Step 2 targeted the health of your heart, lungs and blood vessels by calling on them to "oxygenate" your body through aerobic physical activity. In Step 3, we focus on your muscles and how to make them more toned, strong and supple.

It wasn't long ago that our muscles got a good work-out as a natural consequence of daily living—digging, lifting and moving things manually. But as our lifestyles have changed, our muscles tend to miss out on what they need to keep in shape. Some sports and physically activities such as cycling, rowing and even playing tennis can work our muscles effectively, but in the absence of these muscle-engaging activities you can still keep your muscles strong and functioning at their best by using strength-building exercises.

There are many misconceptions associated with strength-building exercises, more commonly known as *resistance* exercises.

First, most people think it is necessary to join a gym and lift heavy weights. But strength-building exercises can be performed effectively using only your own body weight—you are your own gym!—or simple aids that can be found around your home, such as cans of food or water bottles. You don't need to become a gym junkie to take this third step in the optimal active lifestyle.

A second misconception about resistance exercises is that they are only for young males who are eager to "bulk up" to impress the fairer gender. Instead, it is the opposite demographic—older females—who stand to benefit most from regular resistance exercises. But resistance exercises offer great benefits

I didn't make it to the gym today. That makes five years in a row!

whatever your age or gender. Peak organizations such as the American College of Sports Medicine recommend that people should aim to perform muscle-strengthening exercises two or three days per week.[1] Here are some of the reasons why.

1. Excite your muscles and nerves.

It is good to have strong, toned muscles. Regularly performing resistance exercises can greatly increase strength, which in turn can improve functionality.[2] This can be especially important for elderly people who discover that having the strength to get out of their chair unaided or retrieve items from high cupboards greatly improves their quality of life. Simple abilities make a big difference.

As we age, we tend to experience a loss of muscle tissue—an undesirable condition known as *sarcopenia*—and this contributes to frailty.[3] Sarcopenia is associated not only with a loss in muscle size, but also a loss of muscle quality, as fat and other non-contractile materials infiltrate their way into the muscle.[4] The most important approach for slowing down sarcopenia is to engage in physical activity—and resistance exercises are key.[5]

Improvements in strength occur quickly when someone engages in strength-building exercises for the first time, largely due to positive changes in the nervous system. So resistance exercises are not only good for our muscles, they also make our nerves "come alive." As a result, there is evidence that strength-building exercises also aid brain health and can prevent cognitive decline.[6]

> **WILL RESISTANCE EXERCISES MAKE ME "BIG AND BULKY"?**
> It is a common fear of females that if they perform resistance exercises they will become "big and bulky" but their fear is unfounded. Young males who *want* to experience this effect have to work extremely hard to achieve it and they have vastly greater concentrations of the muscle-building hormone testosterone floating around in their system! Resistance exercises such as those described in this chapter tend to tone a female's muscles, not turn her into a muscle-bound Hercules.

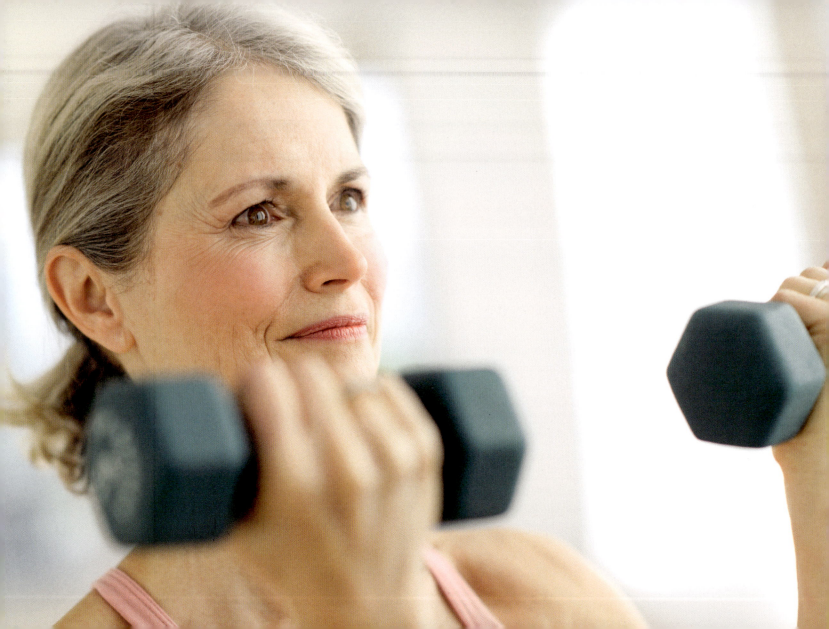

2. Strengthen your bones.

It is not only muscles that grow stronger in response to strength-building exercises. All of the structures that support the muscles also toughen up, including the bones to which the muscles are attached.[7]

Bone strength becomes a major concern as we age because our bones begin to decrease in density after our third decade of life—known as "osteoporosis"—and this speeds up in women after menopause. Weak bones are obviously more susceptible to fracturing, which is a problem especially among the elderly as our sense of balance gets worse as we age, making us more prone to falling. About one-third of adults older than 65 fall at least once per year and many of these falls result in fractures—about 90 per cent of hip fractures are fall-related.[8]

Performed regularly, strength-building exercises are tremendously helpful for reducing fall-related injuries. First, increased muscular strength and control achieved through regular strength training makes falling less likely. Second, by increasing bone density and strength, there is a reduced likelihood of a fracture even if a fall does occur.[9]

Resistance exercises are also highly beneficial for men undergoing hormone therapy for prostate cancer, as they help preserve bone mineral density, which commonly decreases as a side effect of the treatment.[10]

GET BALANCED
Falls in the elderly are now such a concern that the World Health Organization recommends people over the age of 65 years should practise balancing exercises three times a week to improve their balance. A great demonstration of balance exercises can be viewed at the Mayo Clinic: <www.mayoclinic.com/health/balance-exercises/SM00049>.

3. Dial up your metabolism.

Toned muscles burn more energy, so resistance exercises can increase your metabolic rate. This may be extremely important for weight management as your resting metabolic rate—the speed at which your body burns energy when you are relaxed and doing nothing—contributes as much as 70 per cent of your daily energy expenditure.[11] Increasing your metabolic rate by just a few per cent can result in the body burning a lot more energy throughout the day—and night!

If you burn energy at a faster rate, you are less likely to be overweight. It is not surprising that when resistance exercises are combined with "aerobic" activities—as prescribed in the optimal active lifestyle—fat loss is superior to when aerobic activity is performed alone.[12]

SIT-UPS TO LOSE TUMMY FAT?

Even among health experts, there is a common misconception that exercising a particular part of the body will result in fat being lost from that site.[13] For example, individuals will perform sit-ups to lose fat from their abdomen. However, this concept of "spot reduction" is not valid.

Regardless of where it is stored in the body—on the tummy, thighs or bottom—fat is simply the body's excess energy storehouse. Importantly, it is the storehouse for the entire body, not just the nearby muscle. For that reason, the best way to get rid of unwanted fat is to perform exercises that burn lots of energy, involving many muscles working simultaneously as occurs when walking, cycling and swimming.

Performing lots of sit-ups will tone the abdominal muscles but as they are relatively small muscles it will not burn lots of energy. Therefore sit-ups alone are not as effective for weight loss as other large muscle exercises.

A healthy rate of weight loss for most people is about 1 to 2 pounds (0.5 to 1 kilogram) per week.[14] More rapid losses probably mean you are losing muscle as well, which in the long-term can make keeping the weight off more difficult because it may decrease your resting metabolic rate.

4. Control your blood sugar level.

There is excellent evidence to show that regularly performing resistance exercises is extremely beneficial for people with diabetes. Studies have shown improvements in blood-sugar control using resistance training can match—and sometimes exceed—that typically produced by conventional drug treatments.[15] The American Diabetic Association, as well as other peak bodies, recommend that people with diabetes perform resistance exercises two to three times per week.[16]

Resistance exercises are so good for improving blood sugar level control because they place high demands on the muscles, which causes them to increase their ability to uptake glucose for energy. And because resistance exercises only target a portion of the body at a time and are of relatively short duration, they are generally more easily tolerated than other high-intensity activities such as running.[17]

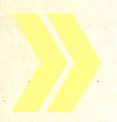

IMPORTANT THINGS TO REMEMBER WHEN PERFORMING RESISTANCE EXERCISES

As resistance exercises are higher intensity, there are a few important safety tips:

1. Do a warm-up activity before getting into the exercises, like a brisk walk or jog, so your muscles are prepared.

2. If you suffer from any musculoskeletal problems that may be aggravated by the exercises or you experience any unusual pain, don't perform that exercise without seeking expert advice. If you perform resistance exercises vigorously, it is normal to experience a "burning" sensation in the muscle due to the production of "lactic acid." Lactic acid does not cause any long-term harm to the muscle and the burning sensation should quickly ease as soon as you cease the exercise.

3. When performing resistance exercises, don't forget to breathe. A good technique is to inhale on the count of three during the lowering phase of the exercise, and exhale on the account of two during the lifting phase.

4. When performing the exercises keep your lower back in a stable, neutral position—don't let it bend unnaturally and keep it steady. Using your stomach muscles to pull your belly button "up and in"—commonly referred to as "activating your core"—can help support your spine.

Oh, the pain! There are two types of muscle soreness related to resistance exercises. The first is that experienced while performing the exercise—often described as a burning sensation—that quickly relieves as soon as the exercise is stopped. The second type of soreness is more mysterious as it presents as "stiffness" one or even two days after.

The exact reason for this soreness—referred to as "delayed-onset muscle soreness" (DOMS)—is not completely understood. However, researchers have determined that lifting a heavy weight does not cause DOMS near as much as lowering the weight back down.[18] Similarly, walking downhill causes more DOMS than walking uphill. Essentially DOMS is provoked when muscle contracts while lengthening as compared to shortening. DOMS is nothing to worry about—as long as it subsides over the course of a few days—and it should fade as you become more accustomed to resistance exercise.

Take a breath! When lifting heavy weights, weightlifters often perform a technique known as the "valsalva maneuver" in which they tense their abdominal muscles and hold their breath—it is a bit like "grunting" without letting any air out of your lungs! The valsalva maneuver can be extremely dangerous if you are not accustomed to it as it causes your blood pressure to skyrocket. Weightlifters have recorded blood pressures as high as 480 (systolic) over 350 (diastolic) mmHg while performing the valsalva maneuver.[19] But for the rest of us—don't forget to breathe!

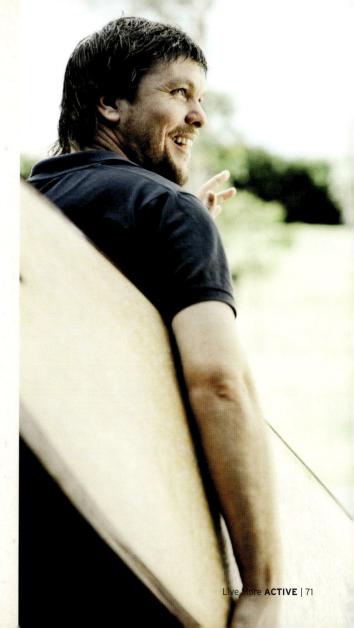

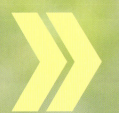

Muscle Action categories

There are many different types of resistance exercises but some of those performed in gyms are quite unusual and do not mimic any action typically performed in "real life." For this reason, there is increasing emphasis on "functional exercises" that simulate the kind of movements we might do in our daily living. Shown below are functional exercises grouped under four "Muscle Action" categories:

> Arms—pushing out
> Arms—pulling in
> Trunk bending
> Legs squatting

For each category, easy through to more challenging exercises are explained and illustrated (and also demonstrated in the DVD that accompanies this book). For the exercises requiring weights, food cans or water bottles (filled with water or sand to the desired weight) can be used.

The effect of a resistance-training program is determined largely by the difficulty of the exercise for you and the associated number of *repetitions* you can perform. As a guide, using a resistance or performing an exercise that you can only do for six to 12 repetitions, tends to cause a muscle to grow in strength and size (an increase in muscle size is referred to as "muscular hypertrophy"). Using resistances that you can perform more than 12 times tends to cause muscle toning and improve muscular endurance.[20] When doing resistance exercises, the last few repetitions should be a bit of a struggle, as this causes the muscles to respond and improve.

For most people, aiming for a level of exercise to perform three "sets" of 12 repetitions, with about a two-minute rest between, is a good target.[21] This will offer great all-round benefits. Performing three sets of each exercise is about 40 per cent more effective at improving muscular strength than performing just one set, but when you are first starting out, just one set still produces good improvement.[22]

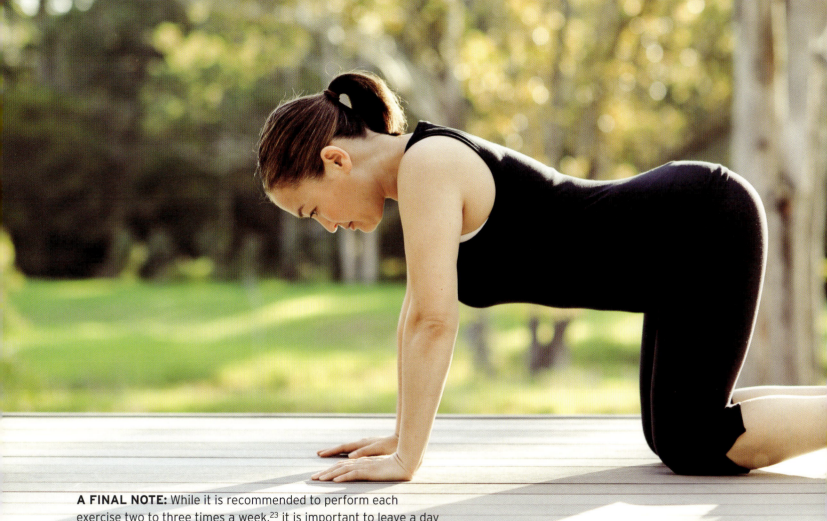

A FINAL NOTE: While it is recommended to perform each exercise two to three times a week,[23] it is important to leave a day or two between so the muscles get plenty of time to recover.

Here are a variety of exercises for each of the four Muscle Action categories listed on page 72.

Muscle Action Category 1: *Arms-pushing out*

These exercises target the muscles of the chest (pectoralis), shoulder (deltoids) and back of the arm (triceps)

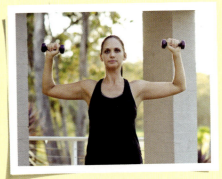

Easy:
SHOULDER PRESS

Start in a standing position with the hands at shoulder height. Be sure to activate your core muscles.

Extend your arms above your head, then return to the starting position.

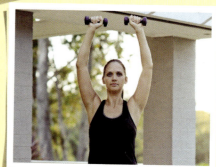

LATERAL RAISE

Start with your arms by your side in a standing position.

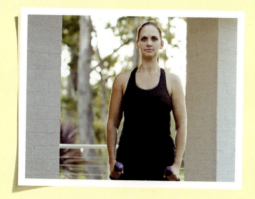 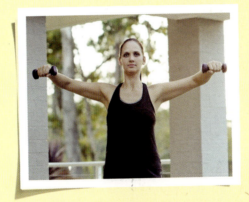

With a slight bend in your arms and palms facing down, raise your arms to the side. Pause just above shoulder height before returning to the starting position.

Note: To increase the level of difficulty, increase the weight.

STANDING PUSH-UPS

Start in a standing position facing a wall with your feet approximately 2 feet (about 0.5 meters) from the wall. Place your hands at shoulder height and width on the wall.

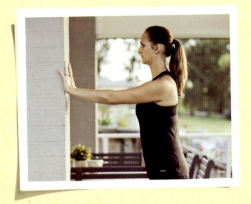 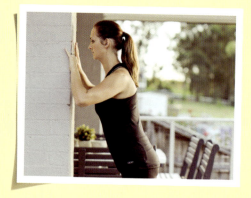

Lean into the wall using your arms, then push back to the starting position.

Be sure to keep your body straight during the action. Activate your core and don't stick your bottom out. Pull your shoulder blades together so you don't slump your shoulders.

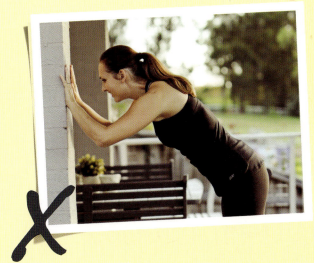

Medium:
DECLINING PUSH-UPS
Adopt the starting position as shown, with your hands on a railing or the corner of a table that won't slide.

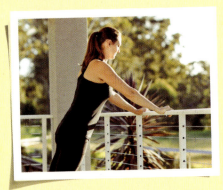 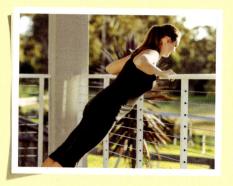

Slowly lower your chest to the railing or table, then push back up to the starting position. Be sure to keep your body straight.

Hard:
FULL PUSH-UPS
With your hands shoulder-width apart and a straight back (activate your core).

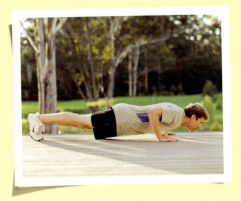
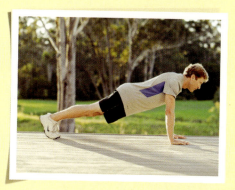

This exercise can be performed with only the feet touching the ground and pivoting from them (as shown) or with the knees touching the ground and pivoting from them (easier version).

Muscle Action Category 2: *Arms-pulling in*

These exercises target the muscles of the upper back (trapezius) and front of the arms (biceps).

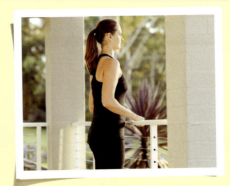

Easy:
STANDING PULL-IN

Stand facing a low wall or post so you can take hold at chest height with your toes touching the base.

Lean back, taking the weight with your arms until they are extended, then pull yourself back to the upright position.

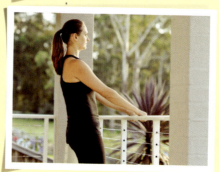

BICEP CURLS

Start with arms by your side, palms facing forward (activate your core).

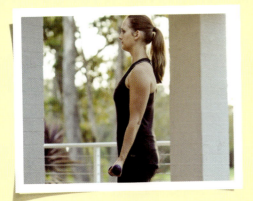 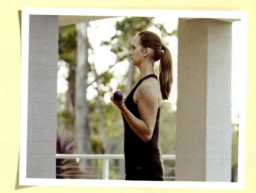

Bending at the elbows, lift the weights to your shoulders, then return to the starting position. You can make this exercise more challenging by increasing the weight.

Medium:
BENT OVER ROW

Adopt the starting position as shown, with a weight in one hand while the other arm acts as a support for your back.

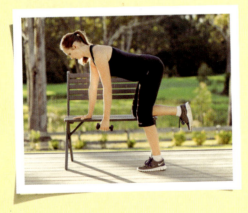
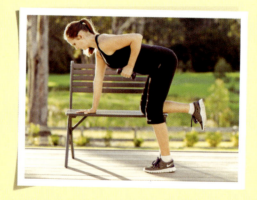

Lift the weight to your armpit, then lower it back to the starting position.

Hard:
To make the exercise more challenging, use a heavier weight.

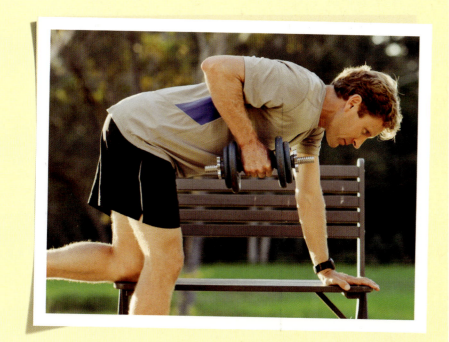

Muscle Action Category 3: *Trunk bending*

These exercises target the abdominal muscles.

Easy:
ABDOMINAL CRUNCH

Adopt the starting position as shown, with your knees bent at least 90°. Activate your core muscles, which should cause your lower back to push into the floor.

Tense your abdominal muscles to slide your fingertips over your knees. You only need to raise your shoulder blades off the floor.

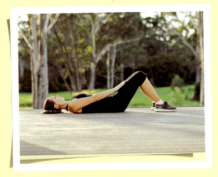

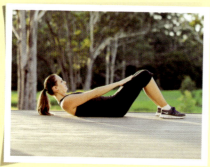

Medium:
BENT LEG CRUNCH
Adopt the position as shown with a 90° bend at your hips and knees. With your arms extended vertically, contract your stomach muscles to raise your shoulders off the floor.

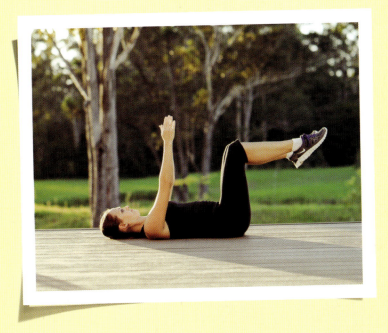

SINGLE LEG EXTENSION

Start with your legs and hips bent at 90°, while pushing your lower back into the floor, activating your core.

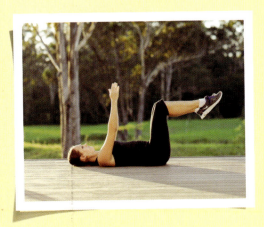 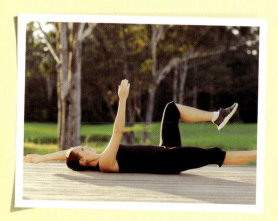

Extend one leg at a time as shown, while keeping your lower back pushed into the floor.

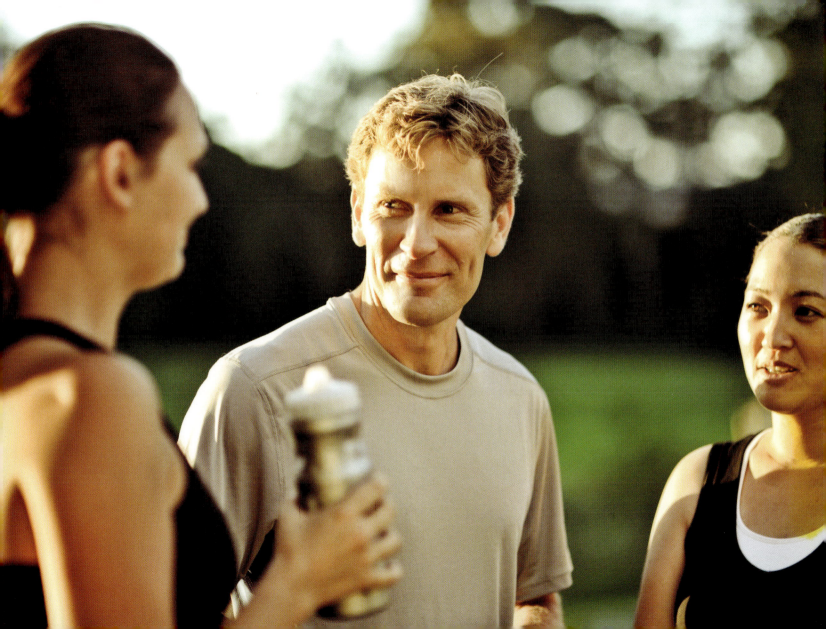

Muscle Action Category 4: *Squatting*

These exercises target the upper leg muscles (quadriceps, gluteals).

Easy:
CHAIR-SUPPORTED SQUATS

Stand behind a chair, holding the top of the backrest for balance.

Keep your back straight as you squat down (pushing your bottom out). Don't bend your knees more than 90°.
Be sure your knees bend in the direction of your toes—don't let them collapse in.

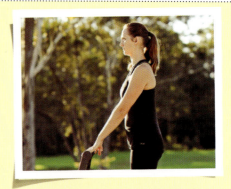

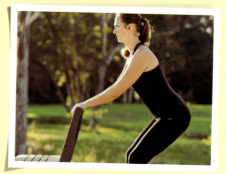

Medium:
SEATED SQUATS

Stand in front of a chair with arms extended to the front.

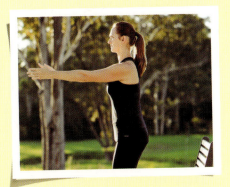 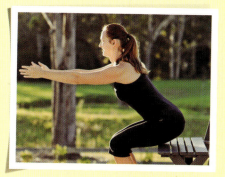

Squat down until your bottom just touches the seat, then raise back up to a standing position. (Keep your back straight and push your bottom out.)

Hard:

To make the exercise more challenging:

1. Hold a weight in your hands (close to your chest) while performing the squat.

2. For a super challenge, try squatting with one leg at a time with the other leg extended in front of you.

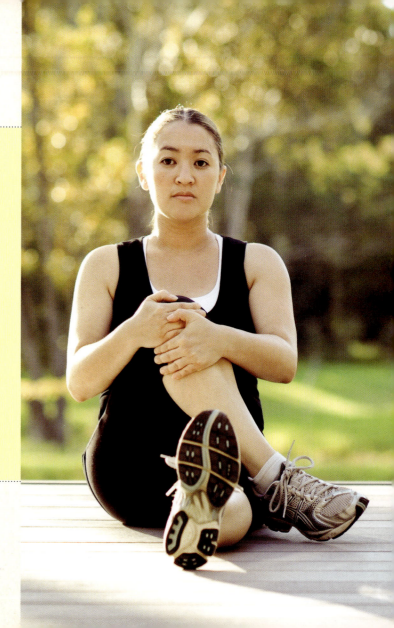

DAY 16

Stretch it out

These resistance exercises are excellent for developing muscular strength, but it is also important to balance this by nurturing the suppleness of our muscles. Suppleness becomes increasingly important as we age, because our body tissue has a tendency to stiffen, which can lead to muscle tension, imbalance and pain. Performing regular stretching exercises can assist in maintaining good flexibility.

It is commonly believed that the best time to stretch is before exercise, but there is no evidence that stretching before exercise decreases the chance of injury. It may even reduce the amount of force your muscles can produce if you are doing high-intensity exercise.[24] It is fine to do light stretches before you get moving but it is not imperative.

Regular stretching not only can make you more supple, it can also help with muscular relaxation and reduce muscle soreness. There is some evidence that stretching actually produces an analgesic—pain-relieving—effect.[25]

Of the various forms of stretching, the safest and easiest is referred to as "static" stretching. A static stretch is one in which the muscle is taken to the end of its range of motion—it should not be painful—and held in that position for 10 to 30 seconds. The stretch is then repeated three or four times. For best results, aim to perform a series of stretching exercises that target different parts of the body two or more times each week.

TRY THESE STRETCHES THAT TARGET MOST OF THE BODY'S MAJOR MUSCLE GROUPS:

1.
2.
3.
4.
5.
6.
7.
8.

1. NECK STRETCHES Keeping your head level, place your finger tips on your chin and gently push your head backwards. Keep your shoulders straight and facing forward, and gently turn your head from side to side. Gently look up and down. Gently tilt your head from side to side.

2. UPPER-BACK STRETCH Extend one arm straight in front, level with your shoulder. Reach across your body and use your other arm to pull it closer to your chest.

3. TRICEP STRETCH Reach your arm vertically upward, then bend the outstretched arm at the elbow so your hand is positioned behind your neck and your elbow is still pointing up. Using the other arm, gently pull the elbow further behind your neck to experience a stretch in the back of your arm.

4. TORSO SIDE STRETCH Adopt the tricep stretch position described above. With feet two shoulder-widths apart, lean away from the side being stretched to experience a stretch down the side of your torso.

5. CAT STRETCH (ABDOMINAL/LOWER BACK) Positioned on your hands and knees, arch your back toward the sky (think angry cat!), then gently transition to arching your back toward the floor (think sway-back donkey).

6. STANDING QUAD STRETCH Holding on to something to steady yourself, bend one leg at the knee until you are holding the instep of your foot with the same-side hand. Gently pull your foot closer to your buttock to increase the stretch. If you can achieve this, gently push your hip forward and knee backwards to further increase the stretch.

7. SEATED HAMSTRING STRETCH In a seated position, extend the leg to be stretched in front of you. Gently reach toward your toes to experience the stretch in the back of your thighs.

8. CALF STRETCH Position yourself on a step while holding on to something to steady yourself. Place the ball of one foot (the side to be stretched) on the step with your heel hanging over the edge. Gently lower your heel down below the step height while keeping your knee straight to feel a stretch in your calf.

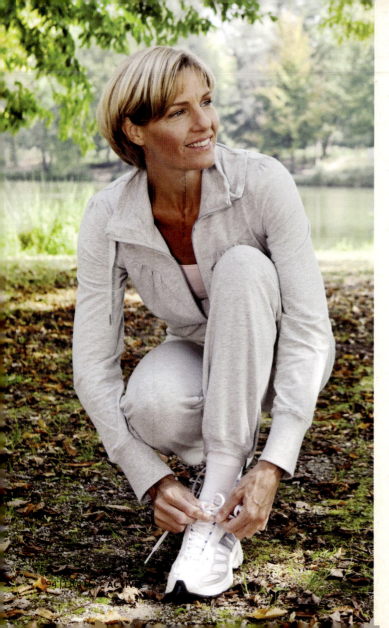

You're all set!

You are now armed with all three steps to achieve the optimal active lifestyle. Implement these principles—Sit less and move more, Oxygenate, Strengthen and stretch (SOS!)—and you are doing everything right in the quest to live more active!

But re-activating your life requires more than just knowing what to do. You need to get your "head-game" working for you. In the final two chapters, we examine two essential components of success.

Chapter Six References

1. N Ratamess, et al (2009), "Progression models in resistance training for healthy adults," *Medicine and Science in Sport and Exercise*, Special Communication, pages 687-708.

2. D Warburton, et al (2006), "Health benefits of physical activity: the evidence," *Canadian Medical Association Journal*, Vol 174 No 6, pages 801-9.

3. F Landi, et al (2010), "Moving against frailty: does physical activity matter?" *Biogerontology*, Vol 11 No 5, pages 537-45.

4. J Ryall, et al (2008), "Cellular and molecular mechanisms underlying age-related skeletal muscle wasting and weakness," *Biogerontology*, Vol 9 No 4, pages 213-28.

5. Landi, op cit.

6. T Liu-Ambrose and M G Donaldson (2009), "Exercise and cognition in older adults: is there a role for resistance training programmes?" *British Journal of Sports Medicine*, Vol 43, pages 25-7.

7. L Nybo, et al (2010), "High-Intensity Training versus Traditional Exercise Interventions for Promoting Health," *Medicine and Science in Sports and Exercise*, Vol 42 No 10, pages 1951-8.

8. N D Carter, et al (2001), "Exercise in the Prevention of Falls in Older People. A Systematic Literature Review Examining the Rationale and the Evidence," *Sports Medicine*, Vol 31 No 6, pages 427-38.

9. J E Layne, et al (1999), "The effects of progressive resistance training on bone density: a review," *Medicine and Science in Sports and Exercise*, Vol 31 No 1, pages 25-30.

10. D A Galvão, et al (2010), "Combined Resistance and Aerobic Exercise Program Reverses Muscle Loss in Men Undergoing Androgen Suppression Therapy for Prostate Cancer Without Bone Metastases: A Randomized Controlled Trial," *Journal of Clinical Oncology*, Vol 28 No 2, pages 340-7.

11. P Stiegler and A Cunliffe (2006), "The Role of Diet and Exercise for the Maintenance of Fat- Free Mass and Resting Metabolic Rate During Weight Loss," *Sports Medicine*, Vol 36 No 3, pages 239-62.

12. J E Donnelly, et al (2009), "Appropriate Physical Activity Intervention Strategies for Weight Loss and Prevention of Weight Regain for Adults: American College of Sports Medicine Position Stand," *Medicine and Science in Sports and Exercise*, Special Communications, pages 459-71.

13. G Egger, et al (2009), "Weight management—Facts and fallacies," *Australian Family Physician*, Vol 38 No 11, pages 921-3.

14. Centers for Disease Control (CDC), "Healthy Weight—it's not a diet, it's a lifestyle!" <http://www.cdc.gov/healthyweight/losing_weight/>.

15. Baker IDI, "Lift for Life," <http://www.liftforlife.com.au>.

16. M D Hordern, et al (2012), "Exercise prescription for patients with type 2 diabetes and pre-diabetes: A position statement Exercise and Sports Science Australia," *Journal of Science and Medicine in Sport*, Vol 15, pages 25-31; R J Sigal, et al (2006), "Physical Activity/Exercise and Type 2 Diabetes: A consensus statement from the American Diabetes Association," *Diabetes Care*, Vol 29 No 6, pages 1433-8.

17. Hordern, op cit.

18. K Cheung, et al (2003), "Delayed onset muscle soreness: treatment strategies and performance factors," *Sports Medicine*, Vol 33 No 2, pages 145-64.

19. J D MacDougall, et al (1985), "Arterial blood pressure response to heavy resistance exercise," *Journal of Applied Physiology*, Vol 58 No 3, pages 785-90.

20. N A Ratamess, et al (2009), "Progression Models in Resistance Training for Healthy Adults," *Medicine and Science in Sports and Medicine*, Special Communication, pages 687-708.

21. ibid.

22. J Krieger (2010), "Single versus multiple sets of resistance exercise for muscle hypertrophy: a meta-analysis," *Journal of Strength and Conditioning Research*, Vol 24 No 4, pages 1150-9.

23. World Health Organization (2010), "Global recommendations on physical activity for health," <whqlibdoc.who.int/publications/2010/9789241599979_eng.pdf>.

24. I Shrier (2004), "Does Stretching Improve Performance? A Systematic and Critical Review of the Literature," *Clinical Journal of Sport Medicine*, Vol 14 No 5, pages 267-73.

25. I Shrier (2007), "Does stretching help prevent injuries?" in D MacAuley and T M Best (editors), *Evidence-based Sports Medicine* (2nd edition), Blackwell Publishing, Massachusetts.

DAY 17

Chapter Seven

Moving to success

In Chapter 3, we explored how to *discover motivation* and, in Section 2, you identified some good reasons for adopting a more active lifestyle—reasons that engender feelings, both pleasurable and painful. Take a moment to go back and re-read—and re-feel—your reasons why you simply *must* live an active life.

If you are like most people, your list will feature more "pain-avoidance" reasons than "pleasure-achieving" ones. When it comes to doing things you are not thrilled about, punishment is often a more powerful motivator than reward, at least in the short-term. As such, pain can actually serve us well for initial momentum.

But to successfully adopt a new behavior in the long-term—such as becoming more active—you need to find pleasure in it. The behavior-change experts who wrote the book *Change Anything* say that to experience long-term success, you must even learn to *love* it![1]

Learning to love activity and exercise can take time, and requires being intentional about maximizing the pleasure and minimizing the pain associated with doing it. If you find the entire experience unpleasant and unbearable, you probably won't persist with it for long—a pattern you may know only too well.

But if you can learn to love it, it will come easy to you. As pioneer lifestyle medicine researcher Dr Dean Ornish points out, only when people transition from "fear of death to joy of living" does motivation come easily and positive lifestyle choices become sustainable.[2]

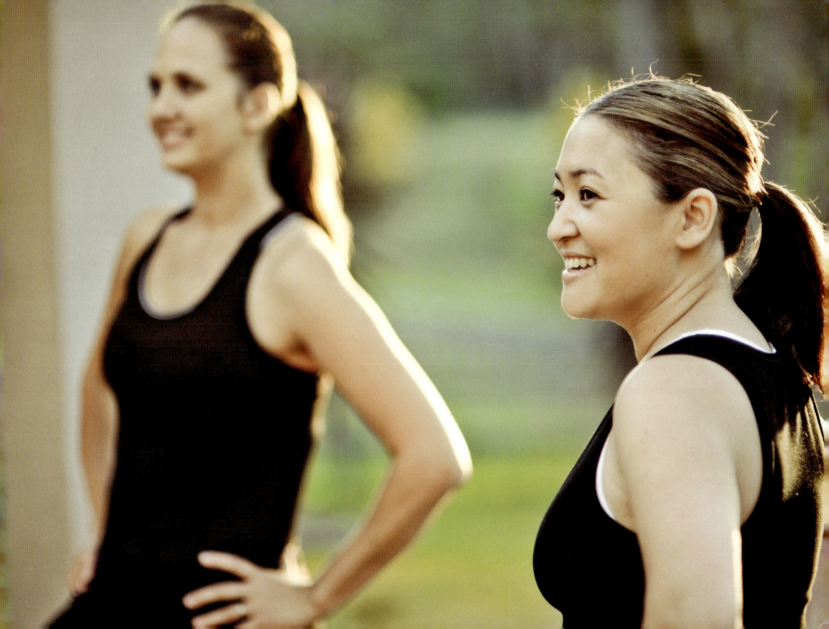

So let's explore strategies that can greatly increase your chance of finding genuine joy in being physically active, including getting your inside and outside world working for you. Get them both on your side and you increase your chance of success by 1000 per cent![3]

Ready, set, . . . slow

One reason so many people fail to stick with an exercise program is because they want instant results, they go too hard, too fast. Perhaps you already know from past experience that this approach equals pain and discomfort, and soon leads to discarding the idea of exercise.

Natural processes take time. I once had a man ask how he could lose 50 pounds (24 kilograms) in eight weeks as he had a class reunion to attend and he wanted to look like his former self. Already knowing the answer, I asked him if he'd gained all that weight in the previous eight weeks. We can't expect to undo in a few days or weeks the result of years of neglect.

The great news is we can experience incredible transformation, but we need to acknowledge and recognize that it takes time, and approach it with this in mind. When it comes to becoming more physically active, our best hope of persisting involves starting slowly and building slowly, which is exactly the approach I have outlined in Section 2 as I have journeyed you toward the optimal active lifestyle.

Some benefits can come quickly—like feeling stronger and more energetic—but others take more time. For example, as we have seen, weight loss *should* take time—a loss of more than about 2 pounds (1 kilogram) per week is not ideal (in the first week or so, it is OK to lose slightly more), as it probably means you are also losing muscle,[4] which will actually make it harder for you keep body fat off in the long-term.

Anything new can take time to get used to but don't make it more unpleasant than it needs to be. Start slow, so you can finish strong. Make like a tortoise, not a hare. Be patient—and the benefits and joys of an active lifestyle will come.

Making your *inside* world work for you.

The ancient philosopher Plato knew what he was talking about when he urged that his followers should "Know thyself." Too often, *we* get in the way of things that are best for us. By understanding how we tick, we can set ourselves up for success. So here are some questions you should consider in order to get your inside world working for you as you move toward the optimal active lifestyle.

Do you have a knowledge gap?

Education changes the way you think, which changes the way you feel, which changes the way you behave. For this reason, education makes more difference than you realize.

As we don't know what we don't know, filling a knowledge gap is inherently difficult. The solution is to seek out good education that identifies for us what we need to know and then teaches it to us. I have designed this book to fill knowledge gaps you may have with regard to living more active but if questions or concerns remain, be sure to seek out the answers.

Story: I was once approached by a man who thanked me for helping him lose 22 pounds (10 kilograms). I was taken aback because I couldn't recall ever meeting him. He explained that he attended a seminar I presented a year earlier and one point struck him. I had explained that it takes about 45 minutes of brisk walking to burn off the calories in one 24-ounce (600-milliliter) bottle of soda. "That fact really struck me as I was drinking several bottles a day," he explained. Learning this single piece of information was all it took for him to switch from soft drink to cold water—and the result was significant weight loss.

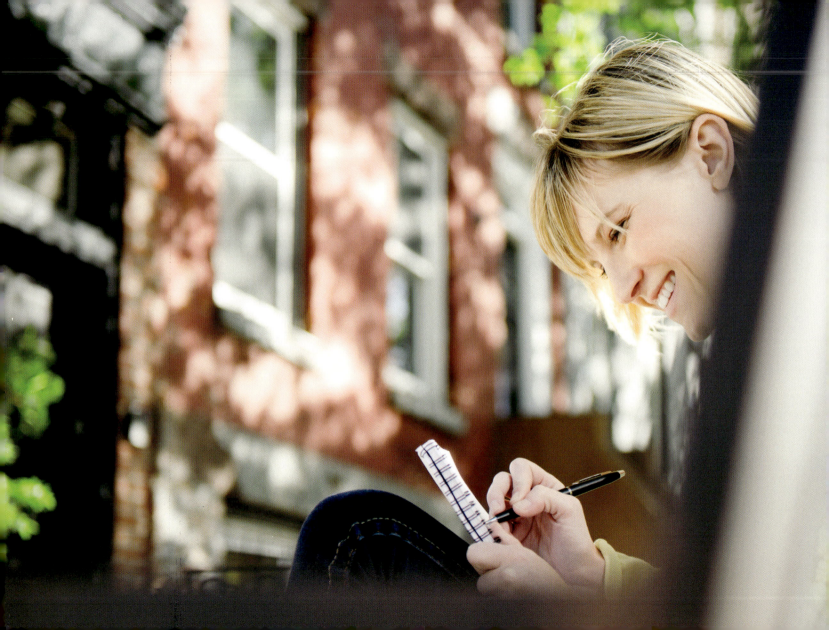

DAY 18

Are you are task-oriented?

Upon opening your eyes in the morning, does your brain instantly begin to create a "to do" list for the day? Do you gain a sense of satisfaction every time you tick an item off your list, but feel glum if too many unchecked items remain at the end of the day? If you can identify, you are a task-oriented individual, so be sure to put "Exercise" as one of the items on your daily to-do list.

Task-orientated individuals—and even many of those who are not—benefit from having a goal to work toward. Goal setting involves "beginning with the end in mind"—one of the seven habits of highly effective people identified by Dr Stephen Covey.[5] Goals can give you something to direct your attention to, energize your level of engagement and commitment, increase your persistence in the face of adversity, and give you a sense of satisfaction when you attain them.[6]

When setting goals, it is best to apply the SMART principle.[7] SMART goals are:

Specific: Goals need to be specific if they are to offer us clear direction. Having a vague goal like "I want to improve my health" is not as motivating as "I want to lose 5 per cent of my body weight."

Measurable: Choosing a goal that has a measureable outcome is more likely to create a higher level of engagement with an action plan than something that can't be clearly measured. As with the examples above, "Losing 5 per cent of my body weight" sets a clear target, whereas "Improving my health" is more difficult to judge in the absence of some quantifiable measures.

Achievable: "I want to go to the Olympics!"—while this might be an achievable goal for some, it is too ambitious for most of us. Challenging goals can be great, but if they are unattainable, we set ourselves up for failure and dissatisfaction, which is extremely demotivating. Choose goals that will stretch you, but not break you.

Relevant: The goals we set for ourselves need to be worthwhile and meaningful, as well as relevant to what we are trying to achieve.

Timely: One of the greatest causes of procrastination is the "one day" mentality: "I will get fitter—one day" or "One day I will start eating better." For goals to be most helpful, they need to be time-framed to create a sense of urgency and help structure a plan to achieve them. It is good to set both short-term and long-term goals that give us something to aim for yearly. Short-term goals can be stepping-stones to encourage us on our journey toward our long-term goals.

In Section 2 (Day 18), you will be guided through a SMART goal-setting exercise.

The landmark study by the Diabetes Prevention Program Research Group set two goals for the study participants: lose 7 per cent of your body weight and perform 150 minutes of moderate-intensity physical activity per week. Those who achieved these goals were half as likely to develop diabetes than those who were put on medication.[8]

Story: David Knight certainly activated his life. Weighing in at around 280 pounds (126 kilograms), he was inspired by the story of John Maclean (see page 55) to try a triathlon. When I met David, he had shed nearly 90 pounds (40 kilograms) and was full of energy as he geared up for his fifth Ironman triathlon. As a fundraiser for John Maclean's foundation, he decided to get sponsorship to do as many sit-ups as he could after completing the event. How many sit-ups can a person do after swimming 2.4 miles (3.8 kilometers), riding 110 miles (180 kilometers) and running 26 miles (42 kilometers)? Given that some sponsors committed $5 per sit-up, they probably figured not many. Imagine their surprise to learn David performed 1125 sit-ups! Talk about the power of worthy goals to motivate![9]

Are you competitive?

Some people thrive on competition. If you do, use competitive situations to fuel your motivation. Competition often inspires our best efforts. You can compete against yourself—by trying to better your efforts—or others—by joining with others who also enjoy competition. But here's a tip from one who is naturally competitive: resist the urge to compete against those who aren't, they don't like it!

Are you an introvert or extrovert?

This question is not the same as, "Are you confident in front of large groups and the life of the party or shy and reclusive?" For example, many professional comedians are introverts. Whether you are an introvert or extrovert relates to where you get your energy. Extroverts come alive by spending time with other people, whereas introverts recharge by inhabiting their own headspace.

If you are an extrovert, exercise with others—it will make it more pleasurable. Plan to be active with a friend or get involved with a sporting team or activity group, such as a hiking club. For extroverts, always exercising alone can make it feel like a punishment—perhaps like you have been sent to sit in the corner by yourself for being naughty!

On the other hand, introverts might discover greater joys from exercising alone. While I enjoy exercising with others, as an introvert, I also cherish the solitary time that exercise affords me and I feel rejuvenated by it. Most of my good ideas come while I exercise alone with my thoughts.

Are you an introvert or extrovert? To maximize your exercise pleasure, structure your active time accordingly.

DAY 19

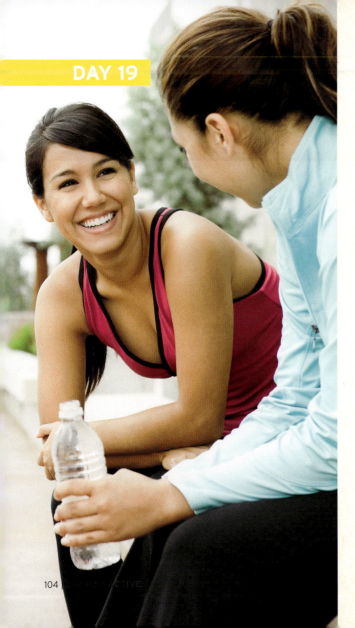

Do you enjoy structure or variety?

Some people love routine, whereas others tire quickly of it. I can't stand to do the same-old day-in-day-out, so I have many physical pursuits I enjoy and I mix it up from day to day. By contrast, I have a friend who loves to do the same thing at the same time each day. As best as you are able, go with what works for you, although there are a couple of important points to consider:

❯ Having a regimented *time* when you exercise is generally best because you have more chance of forming a habit. But if you detest structure or your schedule varies from day to day, be sure to make being physically active a priority by planning ahead. Knowing the night before when you will fit exercise into the next day greatly increases your chances of following through and doing it. And if your best intentions are overtaken by the business of the day, seize any free moments to do something active. Anything is better than nothing.

❯ Even if you are extremely regimented, it is still a good idea to vary the *type* of exercise you perform. I often have people comment that when they first start exercising they notice big improvements but, after a few months, the improvements plateau. The reason for this is that once your body has adapted to the challenges of the exercise you perform, there is no reason for it to make further improvements. To keep the improvements coming, you need to mix up your exercises—this can be as simple as walking a different route or performing different types of resistance exercises.

Are other lifestyle practices making it harder to be physically active?

Other lifestyle practices can cause you to feel a lot less like being active and make it harder to activate your life for good. These include smoking, poor diet and inadequate sleep. While much can be said about these topics, here are a couple of noteworthy points:

Smoking is still one of the leading causes of death and disability in many countries. Every cigarette you smoke robs you of life. If you are smoker, today is a great day to quit, so make contact with your local stop-smoking support program and give up for good. It is amazing how quickly the body begins to heal itself and rediscover life when its owner quits smoking.

Diet and exercise go hand in hand. When you are active, your blood flows more freely around your body—bringing with it life-giving nutrients—but our diet can impede that flow:

› Big meals cause a surge of blood to your gastro-intestinal tract to aid with digestion, so there is less blood available for active muscles. This is why your body tries to deter you from exercising after a large meal by causing you to feel sleepy or making you feel uncomfortable if you do try to do something active, like causing the exercise-related tummy pain known as the "stitch." The lesson: Don't eat a big meal shortly before you exercise or it will be less pleasurable.

› Fatty foods and dehydration can cause your blood to become "thicker" so it doesn't flow as easily. When this occurs, we feel sluggish and exercise is less pleasurable. Therefore, avoid fatty foods, especially before exercising—and be sure to drink eight glasses of water a day.

Sleep is essential for you to function at your best and everything is harder, more arduous and less pleasurable when you are tired. Most people require seven to eight hours sleep each night, so make that a priority. Moreover, if you are not a morning person, don't get up early to exercise—if you can exercise at another time of day. Exercising first thing in the morning is great as it gets it done, but if you are an "owl" rather than a "lark," exercising in the morning is not going to help you love it.

DAY 20

Making your *outside* world work for you.

Even if you have your inside world working for you, outside forces can make or break your resolve to follow through on living more active, as well as many other positive lifestyle choices. These outside forces include the social environment you are immersed in and your physical surroundings. Making your outside world work for you starts with being aware of their potency to influence your behavior.

"I'll get by with a little help from my friends."

The people we associate with and spend time with can have a tremendous impact on our health, as evidenced by a fascinating Harvard study.[10] The researchers tracked more than 12,000 individuals for about 30 years and found that an individual's likelihood of becoming obese increased by 171 per cent if he or she had a friend who became obese. Interestingly, if an individual's spouse became obese, the chance of them becoming obese increased by only 37 per cent. This suggests that our friends may have a greater influence on our lifestyle habits than our spouse! Think twice before praying, "If I can't be thin, at least make my friends fat"—you will probably go with them.

The researchers went on to discover that in social networks, an individual who gains weight increases the chance—by about 10 per cent—that the friends of their friends—three degrees of separation—will also gain weight. And the same was found for happiness: happy people infectiously spread their joy up to three degrees of separation.[11]

Like obesity and happiness, physical activity is socially contagious. If you associate with active people, you are more likely to find yourself participating in active pursuits, without even thinking about it. Conversely, if you spend all your time with people whose greatest joy in life is sitting on the sofa chugging down tubs of ice cream, there is a good chance you will soon be sitting beside them with a spoon in your hand. It is easy to adopt the lifestyle habits of those we spend time with, whether they be good or bad.

The take-away message: In the pursuit of living more active, it helps to seek out positive influences—or better still, be one. By associating with individuals who have succeeded in activating their lives, you can learn their secrets. Success leaves clues.

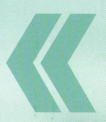

Story: I once ran a marathon. It remains the longest 2 hours, 52 minutes and 43 seconds of my life! I entered the event under-prepared and by the 20-mile (32-kilometer) mark, it felt like my wheels were about to fall off. But I discovered that if I ran beside someone who looked relaxed and fresh, I too began to feel more relaxed and fresh. On the other hand, if I ran beside someone who looked as tired as I felt—even though they were going the same speed as the "fresh" ones—I began to feel all the more exhausted. I was reminded that day that we tend to assimilate to those with whom we associate.

Because social support is so important to facilitating behavior change, I encouraged you in the introduction of this book to team up with others for this journey toward the optimal active lifestyle. If you haven't acted on this advice yet, make every effort to. Teaming with others creates accountability, which can be highly motivating. Knowing that an exercise partner will be waiting for you, greatly increases the likelihood you will show up.

Even if you can't arrange to exercise with a partner, a friend can still keep you accountable by keeping track of how you are going and giving you a prod, if required. Obviously, it needs to be someone you respect and not someone you feel comfortable telling to mind their own business. Having someone keep you honest can make a world of difference to your motivation and physical activity adherence.

So open your eyes to the social forces around you and how they may help or hinder your journey toward the optimal active lifestyle. Make every effort to associate with people who model good choices, hold you accountable, offer good advice and cheer you on. After all, we all need a cheer squad in life!

Story: Wendy struggled to find any consistency when it came to exercising until she teamed up with a couple of friends who were in a similar situation to her. Being a mom with small children meant that getting out of the house for anything other than the absolutely essential was avoided. But when one of the women from her local mothers' group suggested they get together to push prams three mornings a week, Wendy agreed to join in. Wendy discovered many positives came from her morning pram push. First, she felt good for the physical activity. Second, it seemed to do her children wonders to be outside for a while. But most importantly, Wendy felt recharged as a result of the social contact. Being an extrovert, Wendy was fed by associating with other *adults*—and as a result it took something serious to stop her showing up three times a week.

Physical environment

Despite the best of intentions to go walking in the evening, the couch in Jenny's living room would engulf her after dinner and she remained trapped until bedtime. Her nemesis was the TV set. Recognizing her weakness, Jenny moved the TV into a spare room where the only seat belonged to an exercise bike. Jenny gave herself permission to watch as much TV as she liked, on the condition that her legs had to be turning over the cranks. Even though she didn't set a cracking pace, it was activity nonetheless. As we have seen, every bit counts.

But Jenny found this simple re-engineering of her environment not only made her more active, she watched less TV—the bike seat wasn't as comfortable as the couch! With more time on her hands, Jenny found herself becoming more productive all round.

Jenny's story is just one example of how modifying your physical environment can simply but powerfully facilitate behavior change. There are many other ways in which we can force or enable ourselves to move more by rearranging or modifying our space.

Andrew's activity levels substantially increased after he set up a volleyball net on a patch of grass at his worksite—he was also instrumental in encouraging several of his co-workers to be more active as well. In my street, a neighbor showed initiative and mounted a basketball ring on a telegraph pole. The result has been a regular gathering of kids—and parents—shooting hoops and interacting. It's a fantastic asset to our neighborhood!

Health policy makers are becoming only too aware of the importance of creating environments that provide opportunities for people to be active. For example, governments are now taking seriously the need to resource communities with infrastructure conducive to active transport[12] and to create safe and accessible cycle-ways and footpaths. Not only is this a "greener" way to go, it can help eliminate a number of problems large cities face, including traffic congestion, air pollution, greenhouse emissions, noise pollution, and the need for the enormous amount of space required to store, drive and park motor vehicles. Some major cities, such as Paris, have installed easy-to-use bike-hire facilities throughout the city so people can get around under their own steam. It is great for public health, as well as for lessening traffic congestion and pollution.

Be aware of the influence your current physical surroundings are having on your level of physical activity—or inactivity—and get creative about how you can make changes to set you up to move more (see Section 2 for some tips). Behavior-change experts from the Change Anything Labs in the United States attest that "when you transform your environment from foe to friend, you can make the changes that sometimes seem impossible practically inevitable."[13]

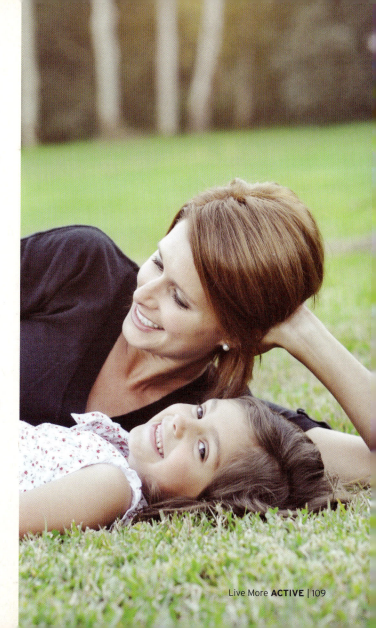

The force of habit

It has been said, "First we make our habits, and then our habits make us" (Charles Noble). The tips we have been exploring aim to make living more active a habit for you, so that in turn that habit can grow you into a fitter, healthier and more lively person. However, habits are sometimes misrepresented. It is sometimes claimed that it takes 28 days to form a habit, but it is possible to form a habit much more quickly—even in an instant. If you are nearly hit by a train as you cross the track because you did not look, you will be certain to look every time from that moment on.

But even those habits that have been with us for many years can also need constant nurturing. And even individuals who are most committed to an active lifestyle have days where they don't feel motivated to move—and sometimes they don't.

It is our daily choices that count. By making positive daily choices, we sustain our habits and those habits create our destiny. As we continue to make positive daily choices, they become easier. As Pythagoras once said, "Choose the best and habit will make it easy and agreeable."

A final point: When it comes to changing a behavior, "relapse" is entirely predictable.[14] As you strive to live more active, there will be times when you will fall back into old sedentary ways. The key is to try not to fall too far or for too long. More importantly, dust yourself off and get back up again. Don't beat yourself up for a failure; the only failure is to not try again.

You're on the journey

To aid your journey toward the optimal active lifestyle, you need to take a good look inside and out. Only by making a careful exploration of who you are and what works for you, as well as by examining the environment around you—both social and physical—can you set yourself up for success. Combined with a good emotive reason(s) for being active (Chapter 3) and laying aside the excuses for not exercising (Chapter 5), you have almost all you require to virtually activate your life for good. But there is one more essential ingredient, without which long-term success is impossible.

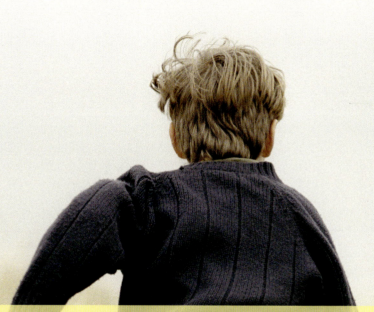

Chapter Seven References

1. K Patterson, et al (2011), *Change Anything: The New Science of Personal Success,* Business Plus.

2. D Ornish (2007), *The Spectrum: A Scientifically Proven Program to Feel Better, Live Longer, Lose Weight, and Gain Health,* Ballantine Books.

3. Patterson, op cit.

4. Mayo Clinic, "Weight loss: 6 strategies for success," <www.mayoclinic.com/health/weight-loss/HQ01625>.

5. S Covey (1989), *The Seven Habits of Highly Effective People,* Simon & Schuster, see "Habit 2: Begin With the End in Mind."

6. E A Locke and G P Latham (2002), "Building a practically useful theory of goal setting and task motivation," *American Psychologist,* Vol 57, pages 705–17.

7. G Doran (1981), "There's a S.M.A.R.T. way to write management's goals and objectives," *Management Review,* Vol 70 No 11, pages 35–6; P Meyer (2003), "What would you do if you knew you couldn't fail? Creating S.M.A.R.T. Goals," *Attitude Is Everything: If You Want to Succeed Above and Beyond,* Meyer Resource Group.

8. The Diabetes Prevention Program Research Group (2002), "Reduction in the incidence of type 2 diabetes with lifestyle intervention or metformin," *New England Journal of Medicine,* Vol 346, pages 393–403.

9. D Morton (2003), "Inspirational Tale: David Knight," *NETWORK for Fitness Professionals,* May edition, pages 18–9.

10. N A Christakis and J H Fowler (2007), "The Spread of Obesity in a Large Social Network over 32 Years," *New England Journal of Medicine,* Vol 357, pages 370–9.

11. J H Fowler and N A Christakis (2008), "Dynamic spread of happiness in a large social network: longitudinal analysis over 20 years in the Framingham Heart Study," *British Medical Journal,* Vol 337, a2338.

12. Australian Local Government Association, Bus Industry Confederation, Cycling Promotion Fund, National heart Foundation of Australia and International Association of Public Transport, "An Australian Vision for Active Transport," < http://www.heartfoundation.org.au/SiteCollection Documents/Active-Vision-for-Active-Transport-Report.pdf>.

13. Patterson, op cit, page 116.

14. J O Prochaska and J C Norcross (2001), "Stages of Change," *Psychotherapy,* Vol 38 No 4, pages 443–8.

Chapter Eight

The power of belief

> Your journey toward the optimal active lifestyle is nearly complete, but there is one more issue we must address if it is to become a permanent part of who you are. Throughout this book, we have dedicated considerable time to exploring the secrets of long-term motivation.
>
> **❯ Chapter 3** developed the notion that we are motivated by feelings, then endeavored to get you emotional about needing to live more active by considering the benefits of doing so and the perils of not.
>
> **❯ Chapter 5** examined the common excuses you might be tempted to use to justify a sedentary existence and responded to them so they can be removed as barriers.
>
> **❯ Chapter 7** looked at setting yourself up for success by identifying what works best for you, enlisting the support of friends, and creating a supportive environment.

The final piece of the puzzle we will explore in this chapter is mostly overlooked, but it is my experience that it is absolutely necessary for long-term behavior change.

As we have learnt, feelings drive our behaviors, but why do different people in similar circumstances feel differently and hence behave differently? To illustrate, consider punctuality. Some individuals are sticklers for time; others are not. If a diligently time-conscious person is running late, they will be overcome with unpleasant feelings, becoming agitated, anxious and frustrated. As a result, they start behaving in ways that will get them to their destination as quickly as possible so they can be relieved of these unpleasant feelings. They might walk or drive faster—maybe even recklessly. On the other hand, a tardy individual generally does not experience such unpleasant feelings when running late—certainly not enough to modify their behavior—so they feel no compulsion to hurry.

But why do some feel stressed, anxious and agitated when running late, while others do not?

At the heart of it, time-aware individuals have certain beliefs about being late, like "It is rude to be late" or "Being late shows you don't care" or "Being late is a poor reflection on you as a person." Those beliefs cause the unpleasant feelings, which, in turn, drive their hurried behaviors.

By contrast, an individual who does not hold such beliefs is not overcome with unpleasant feelings when running late, so does not feel compelled to hurry. An individual with beliefs such as "It is polite to get there a little late in order to give the other person more time to get ready" will actually experience *pleasant* feelings when running late, so are even more inclined to never be on time. Our beliefs serve as the reference for how we think, which influences how we feel, and those feelings drive our behaviors. Or to state it simply, *beliefs drive behavior*.[1]

Whether we realize it or not, we have many beliefs that serve as reference points for how we think, feel and then act. Often we are unaware of the beliefs we hold, but they can have a powerful influence over our life and even act as roadblocks on our journey toward optimal living.

Consider the example of weight loss. Many people lose weight, only to regain it in the following months and years. While physiological explanations have been proposed, psychology plays a huge part. For example, when someone loses a significant amount of body weight but does not change their belief about who they are—the way they see themselves—they tend to gain it back.

The psychology behind this is fascinating. As they start gaining the weight back, it doesn't result in unpleasant feelings—they don't believe they are that thinner person anyway!—so they are unlikely to change their behaviors to keep the weight off. For some individuals, being thinner than what they believe they should be—how they see themselves—can actually cause underlying unpleasant feelings that compel them to behave in ways that sabotage their weight-loss success, until they get back to where they believe they should be. Our beliefs can act like a thermostat setting we keep returning to.

Story: Paul lost nearly 65 pounds (about 30 kilograms) and has kept the weight off for about eight years. He comments that even after losing the weight, it took him some time before he could "look in the mirror and not see a fat person," as he describes it. Changing our beliefs about ourselves—and how we "see" ourselves—can take time, but it is critical for long-term change.

I NEED TO BE ACTIVE. I CAN BE ACTIVE. I DESERVE TO BE ACTIVE AND ENJOY THE BENEFITS.

So what beliefs do you have about physical activity? They have shaped your behaviors in the past and will continue to in the future. If you want to change your ways, you need to embrace three specific beliefs.

I need to be active.

You will be unmotivated to activate your life unless you believe it is imperative that you do so.[2] If you believe an active lifestyle is a non-essential nicety, you will not prioritize it and it will be sacrificed for those things you do value.

First and foremost, you have to believe you need it! This is why from the outset, I have bombarded you with the overwhelming evidence that we are caught up in an inactivity crisis and the damage toll is serious. The intent throughout this book has been to convince you of the fact that you need to move more to live more—and that this is a non-negotiable. Hopefully you are convinced and the belief that you "need to be active" has been firmly ingrained in your brain. But keep reminding yourself of these facts.

I can be active.

Unless you believe change is possible and that you are capable of achieving it, you will clearly have no inclination to strive for it.[3] This belief in your ability to make changes and improve your health is referred to as health-related self-efficacy. Individuals with a high level of self-efficacy are more inclined to initiate better lifestyle choices and persist for longer, and they are less likely to slip back to their old ways.[4] There is truth to the saying, "If you think you can or think you can't, you're right."

> ### THE ONE WHO WINS IS THE ONE WHO EXPECTS TO.
> At the time of his retirement, professor and champion athlete Jack Sinclair reflected on what makes a truly great athlete. He concluded: "In the end it comes down to the great physiological unknown, the psyche; the one who wins is the one who expects to win."[5] This truth applies to many areas of life. We must believe we will be successful—even expect it—before we will become successful.

There are two forces that shape the development of the belief that we can do it: credible sources and personal experience.

Credible sources refer to individuals we find believable as we journey through life, starting predominately with our parents/guardians, but then moving on to our teachers, peers, and finally significant others that may or may not be related or close to us.

It is important to distinguish between "credible" and "incredible" sources. Incredible sources are inspirational, but only credible sources are transformational. For example, watching Olympic athletes perform is inspiring, but it is unlikely to change what we believe we are capable of—after all, they are "incredible." For a source to be "credible" to us, they have to be "like us."

Throughout this book, I have showcased the stories of many ordinary individuals—just like us—who have transformed their life from sloth to active, to reinforce the belief that you too can live more active. They have done it and so can you!

EVERYONE NEEDS A CHEER SQUAD

In a study a colleague and I conducted, we found that when it comes to activating children, parental encouragement is more important that parental modeling. In other words, while it is great for parents to lead by example and be active themselves, the encouragement they give to their children is what really makes the difference to their children's activity levels.[6] Encouraging parents are those who talk with their children about the benefits of being active, act as a taxi (by driving their kids to sport training, etc) and cheer them on. And, of course, it is not only children who need encouragement.

Personal experiences are also incredibly formative of our beliefs. Unfortunately, negative experiences are often more potent than positive ones—you tend to remember the time the dog bit you more vividly than the times you happily patted it. Interestingly, there is a construct called the "Losada Line" which suggests that it takes about three positive experiences to counter one negative.[7]

Hopefully, as you have journeyed through this book, your experience of living more active has been positive. As you move forward, do everything in your power to maximize the positive experiences and minimize the negative ones.

I deserve to be active and enjoy the associated benefits.

The third core belief required for long-term success in the quest to live more often goes unrecognized. It says: "I deserve it."

For many people, credible sources—to them—and unfortunate life experiences have taught them that they do not deserve good things in life. Tragically, they form a belief that they are not valuable or of importance. Individuals who develop such a belief often have no ambition to strive for a better life and, if they find themselves enjoying it, can even sabotage themselves because they do not believe they are entitled to it. Having a healthy sense of your worth as a person is pivotal to living a successful and happy life.

I believe—*I know*—that every person has tremendous value and incredible worth, and deserves a life of health and wholeness. Moreover, worth is not based on what we do, what we own or how broken we might be. You are invaluable just because you are. You deserve an active, vibrant, healthy and happy life.

People blessed with a high self-worth might have no idea what I am talking about here, but if you question your value, you will understand. And you need to change this belief.

1. Tell yourself everyday: "I am of great value. I deserve an abundant, healthy and happy life." Saying it can be the start of believing it. As Muhammad Ali once said, "I am the greatest—I said that even before I knew I was."

2. Find a credible source who will confirm your value. It probably only takes one significant other. Researchers have found that when young people have just one significant adult in their life who accepts them unconditionally, regardless of their physical attractiveness, intelligence or temperamental idiosyncrasies—in other words, a credible source who builds their sense of self-worth—they are far more inclined to grow into confident, competent and caring adults themselves.[8] And the source doesn't even need to be the people around us—many religious people derive their sense of value and worth from their faith.

3. Experience your value by contributing. By giving, we receive—and part of what we receive is an elevated sense of purpose and value. Contributing to a cause bigger than ourselves injects meaning into our life, which allows our life to flourish at the deepest level.[9] There are many ways in which we can contribute and our greatest joys come from sharing our signature strengths—those things that we do best and most naturally. Once identified, get creative about how you can use your strengths to make a positive difference, remembering strength is for service, not status.

The take-away message:

You are a person of value and worth, and you deserve an active, vibrant life and the benefits that accompany it. You must believe this!

PASS IT ON

I would like to leave you with a specific challenge: pass it on. How can you use what you have learned on this "Live More: Active" journey to benefit others? How can you be an agent of change to increase the physical activity levels of others, perhaps in your family, workplace or community? Within your sphere of influence, how can you be part of the solution to the inactivity crisis we are facing? There are many ways to make an active difference in lives of those with whom you associate.

Story: Aileen gained 70 pounds (30 kilograms) during her pregnancy with her first child, and it stuck. Weighing in at just heavier than 220 pounds (100 kilograms), Aileen determined to lose the weight. Five years later, she still has not quite achieved her goal—at 156 pounds (71 kilograms) she still has two pounds to lose to hit her target! However, the most amazing transformation in Aileen is arguably not in her outward appearance, but how she sees herself and the difference she can make. Aileen is now working in the health and fitness industry, helping others discover the same rebirth in health and vitality that she has enjoyed. She also helps run the local community triathlon club. Five years ago, Aileen would have never imagined she would be doing what she is doing today. Why not you?

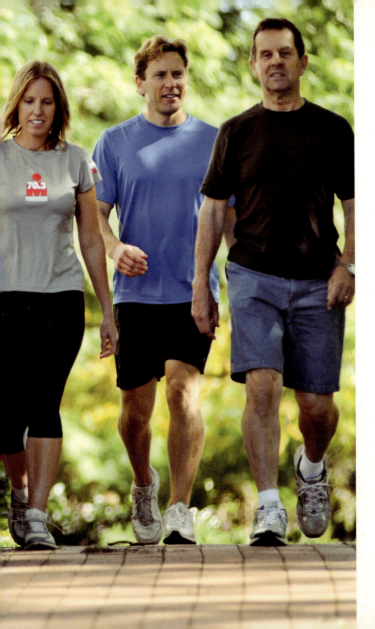

Here are some ideas:

› Start a walking group with friends. Make it an open invitation and spread the word.

› At work, organize the step or VIP challenge described in Section 2 on page 133.

› Start a "walking bus" or "bike bus." In my local community, we have "Friday Ride-day" when children of the area meet together with available adults and ride to and from school. Not only is it great active transport for all involved, it builds community.

› Plan time to participate in active play with your children a couple of times a week. Not only does it model positive behavior, it is great family bonding. When quizzed what children love about their parents or guardians, they most frequently say, "They play with me."

› Lobby your local government to install physical activity opportunities, such as walking or cycling paths or to install publically-accessible exercise equipment.

› Volunteer to coach a local junior sporting team.

Story: Several years ago, my brother and I did some fundraising to create walking trails through the picturesque campus at the university where we work. My house is located near a portion of the trail and, from my back veranda, I can observe how well it is used. It warms my heart to watch individuals, groups and families making their way along the trail. When people are presented with movement opportunities in the form of walking trails and cycling paths, they use them.

I issue this challenge for two reasons:

First, for the benefit of *others*. To combat the inactivity crisis will require many positive agents of change, and I invite you to join me for this most worthwhile cause. You can help save lives.

Second, for the benefit of *you*. The best way to learn anything is to teach it. The best way to make something your own is to become an ambassador for it. "But who am I?" you say. You are perfect for this cause. Don't feel intimidated if you are not yet a picture of health, you will be a "credible source" for others and all the more inspirational.

Becoming an active-life ambassador will result in you seeing yourself differently. It will help consolidate the beliefs: "I need to be active. I can be active. I deserve to be active and enjoy the benefits."

Live your best life.
Live more active!

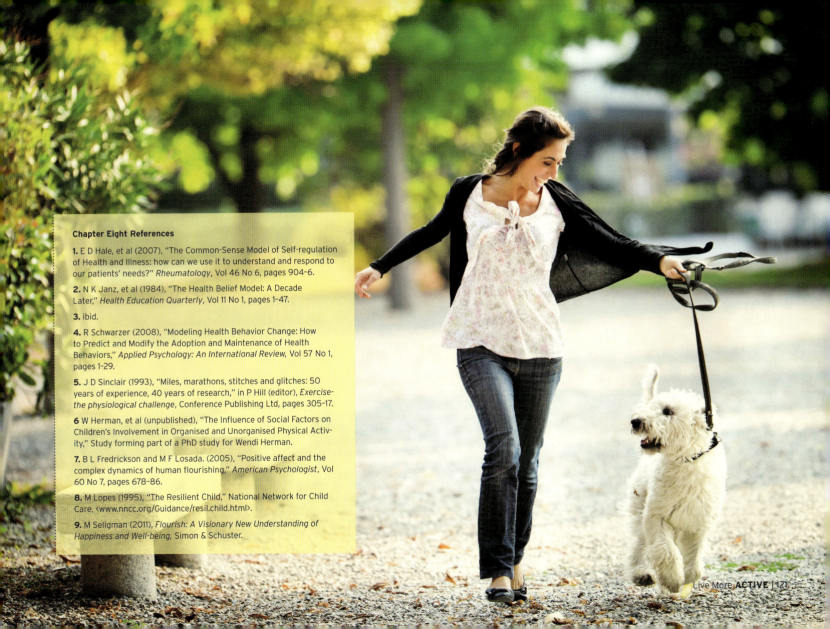

Chapter Eight References

1. E D Hale, et al (2007), "The Common-Sense Model of Self-regulation of Health and Illness: how can we use it to understand and respond to our patients' needs?" *Rheumatology*, Vol 46 No 6, pages 904-6.

2. N K Janz, et al (1984), "The Health Belief Model: A Decade Later," *Health Education Quarterly*, Vol 11 No 1, pages 1-47.

3. ibid.

4. R Schwarzer (2008), "Modeling Health Behavior Change: How to Predict and Modify the Adoption and Maintenance of Health Behaviors," *Applied Psychology: An International Review*, Vol 57 No 1, pages 1-29.

5. J D Sinclair (1993), "Miles, marathons, stitches and glitches: 50 years of experience, 40 years of research," in P Hill (editor), *Exercise- the physiological challenge*, Conference Publishing Ltd, pages 305-17.

6 W Herman, et al (unpublished), "The Influence of Social Factors on Children's Involvement in Organised and Unorganised Physical Activity," Study forming part of a PhD study for Wendi Herman.

7. B L Fredrickson and M F Losada. (2005), "Positive affect and the complex dynamics of human flourishing," *American Psychologist*, Vol 60 No 7, pages 678-86.

8. M Lopes (1995), "The Resilient Child," National Network for Child Care, <www.nncc.org/Guidance/resil.child.html>.

9. M Seligman (2011), *Flourish: A Visionary New Understanding of Happiness and Well-being,* Simon & Schuster.

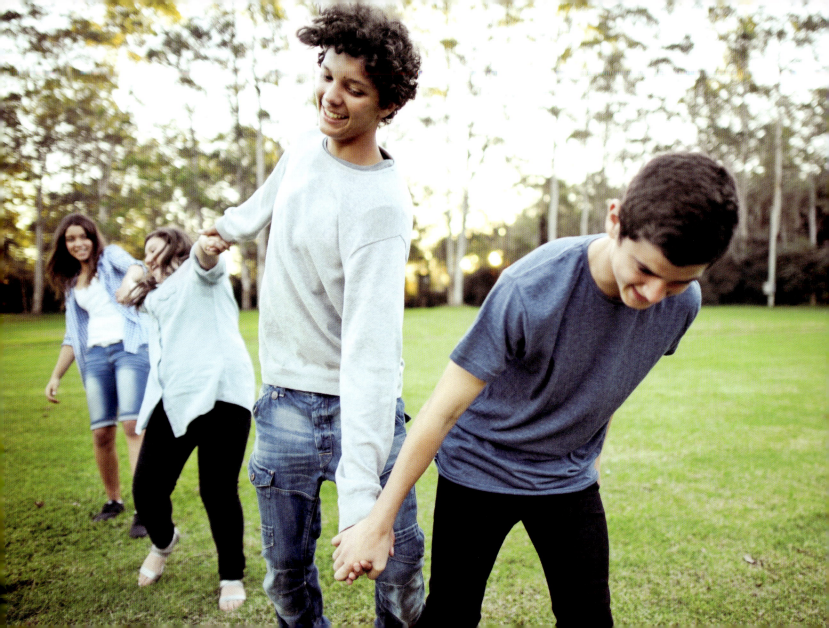

SECTION 2:

Your 21-day activation challenge

In this section, you get to apply to your life what you have learned in Section 1. The content of this book will "come alive" only by road-testing, so I can't urge you strongly enough to give this your best effort.

Consider the next 21 days as a self-experiment. Test it out and see what you discover—it will only be positive. Each day you will be invited to *Learn, Experience and Think.*

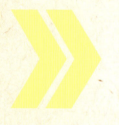

LEARN: Will involve reading a segment from Section 1. If you have already read it, great—but read it again. Repetition is key to learning.

....

EXPERIENCE: Will involve an active challenge for the day.

....

THINK: Will involve you reflecting on what you have learned, as well as how you did on your *Experience* challenge—what worked well and what didn't, and how you could make it work better next time.

There are several ways you can approach this experience, but here is what I suggest as ideal:

> ❯ Set aside a short period of time each evening to read the next day's *Learn* and *Experience* segments. That way you will know what you are up for the next day and can make any necessary preparations.
>
> ❯ The next evening, start with the *Think* segment from the day before to help you appraise how you went during the day. Then read the *Learn* and *Experience* segments for the next day and repeat the pattern.
>
> ❯ Share your learning and experiences with anyone you think might benefit whenever you get the chance!

You will notice that I give you one day off each week, but feel free to do plenty of moving on that day if you wish! Of course, while I have outlined the ideal way to approach this journey, you have the freedom to do it any way that works best for you.

Finally, I want to reinforce what I mentioned at the outset of this book. For best results, embark upon this "Live More: Active" experience with one or more other people. Social support and accountability make a huge difference, so rope in your friend, spouse or workmates. Even discuss your responses to the "Think" questions together. We usually need others to do and be our best.

It's time to get active!

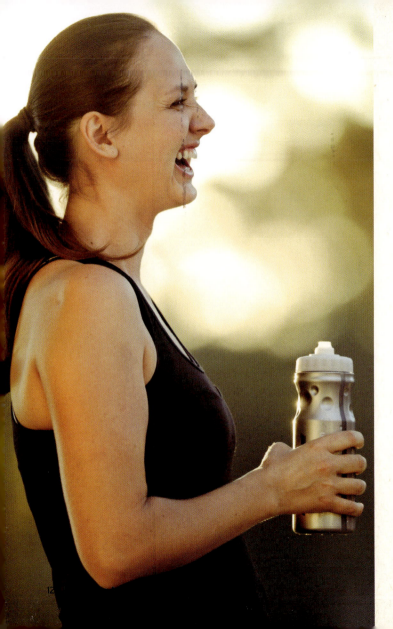

DAY 01

LEARN: Read Chapter 1 "SOS: How to be saved from the inactivity crisis" (pages 6-11).

EXPERIENCE: *Today you have two tasks.*

1. Beg, borrow or buy a pedometer. You are going to need it starting tomorrow. They are easy to come by and can be purchased inexpensively (although beware of the really cheap ones, as they can be unreliable). If you have a smart phone you can also download a pedometer app (I like "Pacer" as it also alerts you when you have not moved in a while). If you already have a pedometer, wear it today but don't try to take any more steps than you would normally—what we are interested in is how active you presently are on a typical day. Record your steps in the first column of the activity log on page 185 (you will learn about the other columns as your *Live More: Active* challenge unfolds).

2. Beginning today, I want you to raise your (water-filled) glass more often! Hydration is paramount for good health and it will become increasingly important as you begin to live more active. Endeavor to drink eight glasses every day. You know if you are hydrated if your urine is clear and odorless—yes, get into the habit of checking! If it is yellow, you are probably dehydrated, so drink up and "don't go for the gold."

Here are some tips for helping you achieve eight glasses per day:

› **Keep a water bottle with you during the day,** perhaps at your desk, in the car or wherever it will be within easy reach. This helps you keep track of how much you've drunk through the day and is a visual reminder.

› **Keep your water cold.** Many people find the taste and refreshing nature of cold water more appealing than room-temperature water.

› **Spice it up.** Some people find the taste of water boring, so try adding a slice of lemon or lime to your water to bring it to life without filling it with calories.

› **Hourly reminder.** Set a reminder on your phone or computer at work to go off every hour to remind you to drink a glass of water.

› **Try drinking a glass of water before each meal.** Meal times work as a good reminder and drinking water helps fill you up, while containing no calories.

› **Start the day hydrated.** Drink two glasses of water every morning after waking up.

› **After going to the bathroom, drink a glass of water.** The "call of nature" provides a good opportunity to stretch your legs and refresh.

THINK:

1. Are you surprised to learn how inactive we have become in recent years? Is it your experience that the world is changing in ways that makes inactivity the default?

....

....

....

2. What areas of your life are you most inactive—work, transportation or recreation? Has this always been the case?

....

....

....

3. Did you get through your eight glasses of water today? Did you feel any different for it?

....

....

....

DAY 02

LEARN: Read Chapter 2 "Step 1: Sit less, move more!" to "Practical Tips for Sitting Less" (pages 12-15).

EXPERIENCE: Your challenge for today is to simply fasten your pedometer and wear it for the day. Try to forget it is there and resist the temptation to look at the screen throughout the day to see how many steps you are up to. Try to do what you would normally do on a typical day—don't consciously modify your behavior to get a better score. The purpose is to get a reference for how many steps you typically take on an average day, before you embarked upon the journey toward the optimal active lifestyle. At the end of the day, note how many steps you took and record it in the activity log on page 185.

THINK:

1. Does it surprise you that "sit time" is an independent risk factor for chronic disease and premature death?

....

....

....

2. Use the table on the following two pages to calculate how much time you spend being sedentary and active on a typical day (tick how you usually spend the indicated time periods and then tally the total at the bottom of the table). Are you surprised by how many hours you are sedentary in a typical 24-hour period?

TIME PERIOD	TYPE OF ACTIVITY				
	Sleeping	Sitting	Light Activities	Moderate Activities	Strenuous Activities
12:00 - 12:30 am					
12:30 - 1:00 am					
1:00 - 1:30 am					
1:30 - 2:00 am					
2:00 - 2:30 am					
2:30 - 3:00 am					
3:00 - 3:30 am					
3:30 - 4:00 am					
4:00 - 4:30 am					
4:30 - 5:00 am					
5:00 - 5:30 am					
5:30 - 6:00 am					
6:00 - 6:30 am					
6:30 - 7:00 am					
7:00 - 7:30 am					
7:30 - 8:00 am					
8:00 - 8:30 am					
8:30 - 9:00 am					
9:00 - 9:30 am					
9:30 - 10:00 am					
10:00 - 10:30 am					
10:30 - 11:00 am					
11:00 - 11:30 am					
11:30 - 12:00 noon					

TIME PERIOD	TYPE OF ACTIVITY				
	Sleeping	Sitting	Light Activities	Moderate Activities	Strenuous Activities
12:00 - 12:30 pm					
12:30 - 1:00 pm					
1:00 - 1:30 pm					
1:30 - 2:00 pm					
2:00 - 2:30 pm					
2:30 - 3:00 pm					
3:00 - 3:30 pm					
3:30 - 4:00 pm					
4:00 - 4:30 pm					
4:30 - 5:00 pm					
5:00 - 5:30 pm					
5:30 - 6:00 pm					
6:00 - 6:30 pm					
6:30 - 7:00 pm					
7:00 - 7:30 pm					
7:30 - 8:00 pm					
8:00 - 8:30 pm					
8:30 - 9:00 pm					
9:00 - 9:30 pm					
9:30 - 10:00 pm					
10:00 - 10:30 pm					
10:30 - 11:00 pm					
11:00 - 11:30 pm					
11:30 - 12:00 midnight					
24 HR TOTAL (remember one tick = ½ an hour)					

DAY 03

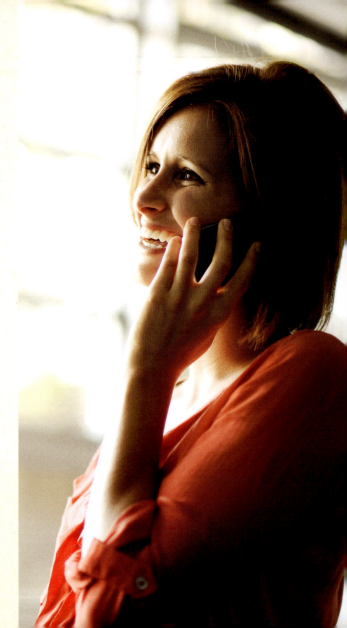

LEARN: Read Chapter 2 "Step it out" (pages 16-17).

EXPERIENCE:

1. Your challenge today is to activate the "3 every 30" principle. Whenever you have been sitting for 30 minutes straight, get on your feet for three minutes. When watching TV, stand up and move about during the commercial breaks between shows. In meetings that you anticipate will drag on for hours, announce before it starts that you are on the "Live More: Active" 21-day challenge and you will be standing for three minutes every half hour as there are great health and concentration benefits. (You might find others standing with you!)

2. Record your number of steps for the day in the activity log on page 185.

THINK:

1. Has willpower failed you in the past? Can you identify with the idea that we do what we do for a feeling? What are some examples?

....

....

....

....

2. How did you go with the "3 every 30" principle? What are some ways you can make this a more permanent part of your lifestyle?

....

....

....

....

DAY 04

LEARN: Read Chapter 3 "Discovering motivation" (pages 18-20).

EXPERIENCE: Today you have two challenges:

1. Take notice of your pedometer. Feel free to check it regularly and stare at it adoringly. Experiment with short excursions, like fetching a drink of water, and take note of how many steps it takes. Record how many steps you took at the end of the day in the activity log on page 185.

2. Identify three things you can commit to for the remainder of this "Live More: Active" challenge—and possibly beyond—that will help you sit less and move more. These might be small things like standing up for the first minute of every phone call or walking on the spot during commercial breaks when watching TV. It is better to make small promises that you will follow through on, rather than grand ones you won't. Keeping promises to yourself builds integrity and self-confidence.

Three things I will commit to doing to sit less and move more:

1. ....

2. ....

3. ....

Write them down somewhere that you can see them and be reminded, or tell someone who can help keep you accountable.

THINK:

1. Did you take more steps today than yesterday because you were more intentional about sitting less and moving more? How close did you come to the target of 10,000 steps? What do you think is a reasonable daily target for you?*

....

....

....

2. How did you go with the three "sit less, move more" strategies you committed to?

....

....

....

* To make counting steps more fun, or to get friends and work colleagues involved with your "Live More: Active" activation, check out <www.10000steps.org.au>. It is free and allows you to keep track of your daily step tally, and do virtual walking challenges based on significant sites around the world.

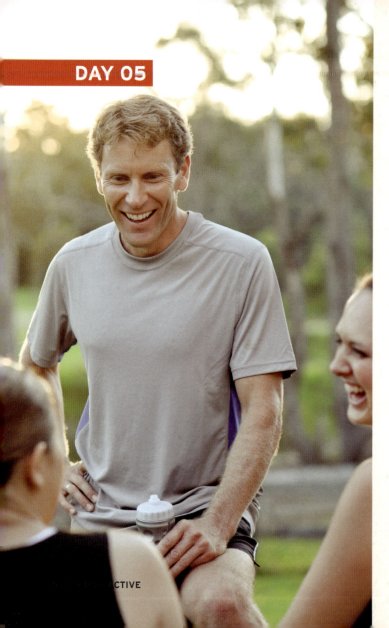

DAY 05

LEARN: Read Chapter 3 "Discovering motivation": "The benefits of living more active," "Live longer" and "Live livelier" (pages 21-28).

EXPERIENCE:

1. Today we turn our attention to the amount of "screen time" you are exposed to. Your challenge is to do something active (such as going for a walk) at a time that you would usually sit in front of a screen (such as watching TV, playing a computer game, working on a computer or surfing the internet). Today, endeavor to swap at least 10 minutes of screen time for activity time.

2. Record how many steps you took for the day and record it in the activity log on page 185, but this time, also convert these steps to Vitality Improvements Points (VIPs).

INTRODUCING VITALITY IMPROVEMENT POINTS (VIPs)

Recording VIPs is simply another way of quantifying how active you are, but it has advantages over step counting, as we will see in the days to come. VIPs will become increasingly important as we progress on the 21-day "Live More: Active" challenge, so now is a good time to learn about them. Converting from steps to VIPs is simple:

1 VIP = 1000 steps

If you achieve 10,000 steps in a day—which is a good goal to have—you achieve 10 VIPs. Hence, 10 VIPs is a great daily target. Therefore, your new mantra is: "Make today a 10!" Of course, you can do more than 10 VIPs if you wish!

As we all have days that are more active and others that are less active, it can be helpful to set a weekly target. A good weekly target is 50 to 70 VIPs. If you can do more, fantastic! If you are not presently up to this level, that is OK too. Do what you can, with the aim to improve on it.

Aim for a weekly target of 50 to 70 VIPs

For best results, try not to get into the habit of achieving your weekly quota of VIPs on the weekend, then not move a muscle during the week. Just like you don't eat all your weekly food on the weekend and expect it to sustain you all week, it is best to spread out your physical activity as well.

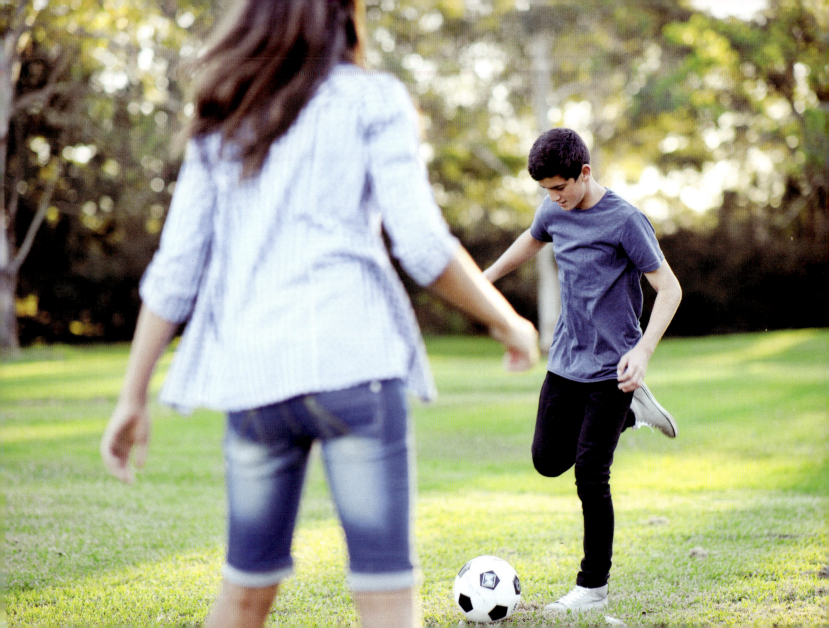

THINK:

1. Do you know someone who died prematurely but might have lived longer if they had lived more active? How does this make you feel? Do you know someone who sufferers from a chronic disease who could benefit from living more active? Why don't you share what you are learning and invite them on the journey with you?

....

....

....

2. Are you sick and tired of being sick and tired? How important is living "livelier" to you? What would you do with more energy?

....

....

....

3. How did you go swapping some screen time with something active? What would it take for you to do it more regularly?

....

....

....

DAY 06

LEARN: Read Chapter 3 "Discovering motivation": "Live leaner" (pages 29-32).

EXPERIENCE:

1. Make an effort today to achieve your personal-best step count (and associated VIP count) for the week. Record your achievement in the activity log on page 185.

2. Calculate your Body Mass Index (BMI).

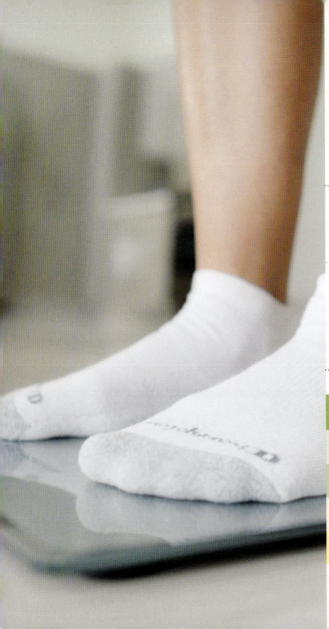

BODY MASS INDEX (BMI)

While it has some limitations, Body Mass Index (BMI) can be a useful tool for assessing where you fall on the healthy weight range. Calculate your BMI to see where you fall:

How to calculate Body Mass Index

$$\text{BMI}_{\text{Imperial}} = \frac{\text{Weight (pounds)}}{\text{Height x height (inches)}} \times 703 = \underline{\qquad}$$

OR

$$\text{BMI}_{\text{Metric}} = \frac{\text{Weight (kg)}}{\text{Height x height (m)}} = \underline{\qquad}$$

BMI	Range of weight
Under 18.5	Underweight
18.5 to 24.9	Normal or healthy weight
25.0 to 29.9	Overweight
Over 30.0	Obese

THINK:

1. What might your future look like if you *don't* follow through and activate your life for good? Identify which of the following risks you most dread, by rating them as indicated:

	Not at all worried								Greatly concerned	
Dying prematurely	1	2	3	4	5	6	7	8	9	10
Suffering from diabetes	1	2	3	4	5	6	7	8	9	10
Suffering from heart disease	1	2	3	4	5	6	7	8	9	10
Suffering from other chronic diseases	1	2	3	4	5	6	7	8	9	10
Becoming frail and less independent	1	2	3	4	5	6	7	8	9	10
Gaining weight	1	2	3	4	5	6	7	8	9	10

Take a moment to reflect on these.

2. What might your future look like if you *do* follow through and activate your life for good? Identify which of the following benefits you would most enjoy, by rating them as indicated:

	Not at all worried								Greatly concerned	
Live longer	1	2	3	4	5	6	7	8	9	10
Live independently to later in life	1	2	3	4	5	6	7	8	9	10
Not being a burden on others	1	2	3	4	5	6	7	8	9	10
More disease resistant	1	2	3	4	5	6	7	8	9	10
More energy	1	2	3	4	5	6	7	8	9	10
Be a good example to others	1	2	3	4	5	6	7	8	9	10
Lose weight	1	2	3	4	5	6	7	8	9	10
Feel better *in* myself	1	2	3	4	5	6	7	8	9	10
Feel better *about* myself	1	2	3	4	5	6	7	8	9	10

Take a moment to reflect on these.

Without emotive reasons for living more active, you are unlikely to follow through long-term. Commit these thoughts and feelings to memory, and remind yourself of them often. Write them out and put them in your wallet or purse. Make them the wallpaper or screen saver on your computer. They will serve you well as you journey toward living more active.

DAY 07
REST

REST DAY!

You have a day off from challenges. Intriguingly, the human body seems to work most effectively on a six-days-on, one-day-off cycle. One day off in seven provides your body with time to rest and restore, which it needs to be at its best.

I am not suggesting you laze around and not move a muscle, in fact you will find it increasingly hard to be completely sedentary as you get into the habit of being active. It is not required but feel free to record how many steps you take (or VIPs) in the activity log on page 185. Enjoy yourself!

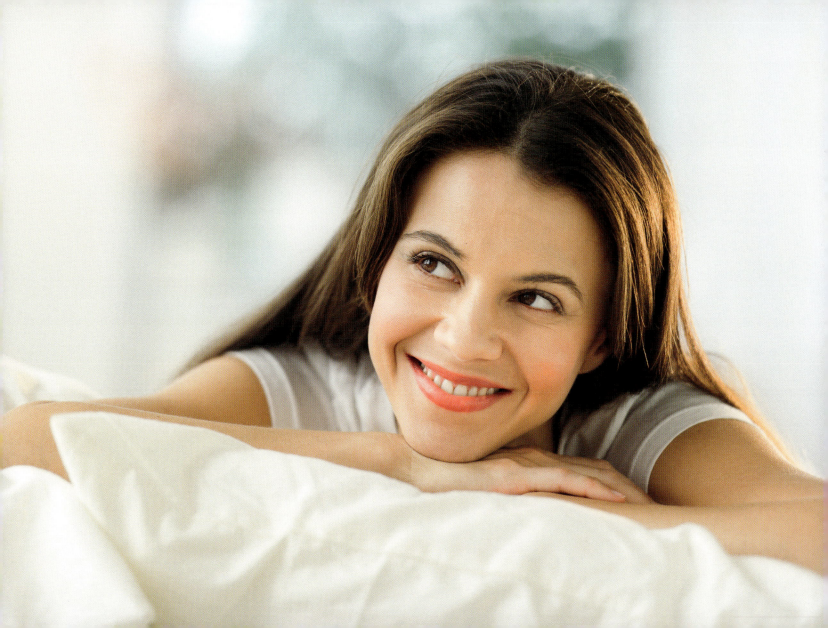

DAY 08

If you do the math, you will realize that to "make today a 10"—achieving 10 VIPs—you will need to perform 50 minutes of moderate-intensity physical activity. This is roughly equivalent to taking 10,000 steps.

LEARN: Read Chapter 4 "Oxygenate" (pages 37-40).

EXPERIENCE:

1. Set aside some time today to explore what "moderate-intensity" physical activity means for you. Put on some comfortable clothing and footwear, and find somewhere you can walk unhindered. Start slowly with a casual stroll and ask yourself, "What would I rate this out of 10 in effort?" Every couple of minutes build up the speed until you would rate the effort as a 3- to 4-out-of-10. Check to see if you could hold a conversation without having to stop between sentences to take an extra breath. Try singing (to yourself) to make sure you can't do it without taking a breather. Once you have found your "moderate-intensity" speed, hold the pace for at least 10 minutes.* See if you can achieve 30 minutes of moderate-intensity physical activity today.

2. Record your steps for the day, converted to VIPs, in the activity log on page 186. Also, let me introduce you to another way of counting VIPs, beyond the "1 VIP = 1000 steps" method. You will find this other method more convenient if you don't have or don't like pedometers, or if you like to perform exercises that pedometers don't count, such as swimming and cycling.

THE "EXERCISE METHOD" FOR COUNTING VIPS

The method is simple. If you can hold your hand on your heart and say you made an effort to "sit less and move more" during the course of the day, you get 5 VIPs. So far so good—but that is where the free ride ends! You have to earn extra VIPs and you are awarded 1 VIP for every 10 minutes of moderate-intensity physical activity you perform. To summarize:

Being intentional about sitting less and moving more = 5 VIPS

Each 10 minutes of moderate-intensity physical activity = 1 VIP

*You can perform this exact same routine for activities other than walking, such as cycling or swimming.

THINK:

1. Is "moderate-intensity" physical activity easier than you imagined? Did you think that you had to go harder to experience great health benefits?

....
....
....
....
....
....
....
....

2. How would you rate your "moderate-intensity" speed?

☐ Very slow stroll   ☐ Slow walk   ☐ Brisk walk   ☐ Fast walk   ☐ Slow jog   ☐ Moderate jog   ☐ Fast jog

DAY 09

LEARN: Read Chapter 4 "Oxygenate": "Get with the beat" (pages 41-43).

EXPERIENCE:

1. Today we continue our exploration of what moderate-intensity physical activity means for you. Yesterday you used subjective measures—judging for yourself how intensely you were going—but today we will use your heart rate as a more objective measure. I should point out that if checking your heart rate doesn't interest you, that's fine, just continue to judge for yourself what constitutes moderate-intensity exercise for you. However, monitoring your heart rate can be helpful for developing a better understanding of your body and how it responds to exercise. So here we go.

You can use a heart-rate monitor for measuring your heart rate, but you can also do this manually, as described below.

Finding a pulse:

You can take your heart rate by feeling your pulse, which is possible where an artery passes close to the surface of the skin. Arteries are the blood vessels that lead directly away from the heart. Every time the heart beats and blood gets forced into them, they bulge slightly and we can feel it as a pulse. You can find a pulse in your wrist (radial pulse), groin, armpit and thumb, but the easiest to locate is in your neck (the carotid pulse). The carotid pulse can be found in the soft spot just to the side of your "Adams apple."

Resting heart rate:

Use your index and middle finger to find your carotid pulse. While sitting in a reclined position or lying down, count how many beats occur in 60 seconds. This is your resting heart rate and it is at its lowest in the early morning when you are well rested.

My resting heart rate = _____ beats per minute

It is fun to keep track of your resting heart rate, as it will often decrease as you get fitter. It is not uncommon for athletes to have resting heart rates in the 40s and former world-champion triathlete, Greg Welsh, had a resting heart rate of only 28 beats per minute!

Maximum heart rate:

Relax, we are not actually going to do this! But you can predict your maximum heart rate using the following equation:

Predicted maximum heart rate = 220 - Your age.

My predicted maximum heart rate = _____ beats per minute

This is only an approximation. There is considerable variation from individual to individual.

Using heart rate to estimate your moderate-intensity zone.

As shown on page 43, you can estimate your moderate-intensity zone by calculating 55 to 70 per cent of your maximum heart rate.

> **Moderate-intensity zone = 0.55 x My predicted maximum heart rate (lower limit)**
>
> **Moderate-intensity zone = 0.70 x My predicted maximum heart rate (upper limit)**
>
> My lower limit   = _____ **beats per minute**
>
> My upper limit   = _____ **beats per minute**

Today, during your activity time, go at an intensity that you would deem "moderate" and take your heart rate. You might find it difficult to locate your pulse and count beats while moving—this is where heart rate monitors are handy—so if you need to, you can pause while you count. So that your heart rate doesn't slow down too much while you are stopped and give you a false measure, only count for 15 seconds, then multiply that 15-second count by four to convert to beats per minute.

2. Record your number of VIPs for the day in the activity log on page 186.

THINK:

1. Is heart-rate monitoring something that interests you or is it too much bother? Why?

....

....

....

....

....

2. If you did try monitoring your heart rate today, did the intensity you judged to be of a "moderate-intensity" fall within your calculated upper and lower heart rate limits?

....

....

....

DAY 10

LEARN: Read Chapter 4 "Oxygenate": "The extra benefits of going vigorous" (pages 44-47).

EXPERIENCE:

1. Today we explore what "vigorous-intensity" physical activity means for you. Of course, you only have to experiment with it if it is something you feel you would like do. There are extra benefits from engaging in vigorous-intensity exercise, as you have already learned, but it is not imperative for good health—moderate-intensity works just great.

If you are up for it, put on some comfortable clothing and footwear, and find somewhere you can exercise unhindered. Build up to your moderate-intensity pace, then start to speed up slowly until you are exercising at a level you would describe as a 5- or 6-out-of-10. You should notice your breathing is considerably elevated and you cannot hold a conversation without taking catch-up breaths between sentences.

There are many health benefits of vigorous-intensity exercise—largely because it "oxygenates" your body so effectively. But there is also a practical benefit: you don't have to do as much of it, so you can achieve your exercise quota more efficiently. While you achieve 1 VIP for every 10 minutes of moderate-intensity physical activity, you only need to perform five minutes of vigorous-intensity exercise to achieve 1 VIP. Therefore, you can achieve your daily VIPs by the "steps method" or the "exercise method":

STEPS METHOD:

1000 steps = 1 VIP

EXERCISE METHOD:

Being intentional about sitting less and moving more = 5 VIPs

+ 10 minutes of moderate-intensity physical activity = 1 VIP

and/or 5 minutes of vigorous-intensity physical activity = 1 VIP

Before you rush out and get vigorous, you should do so with caution as it places higher demands on your cardio-respiratory system. To make sure you are safe to proceed, answer the questions on page 46 (from Section 1). If you answer yes to any of these questions, visit your doctor to get the "all clear" before you start.

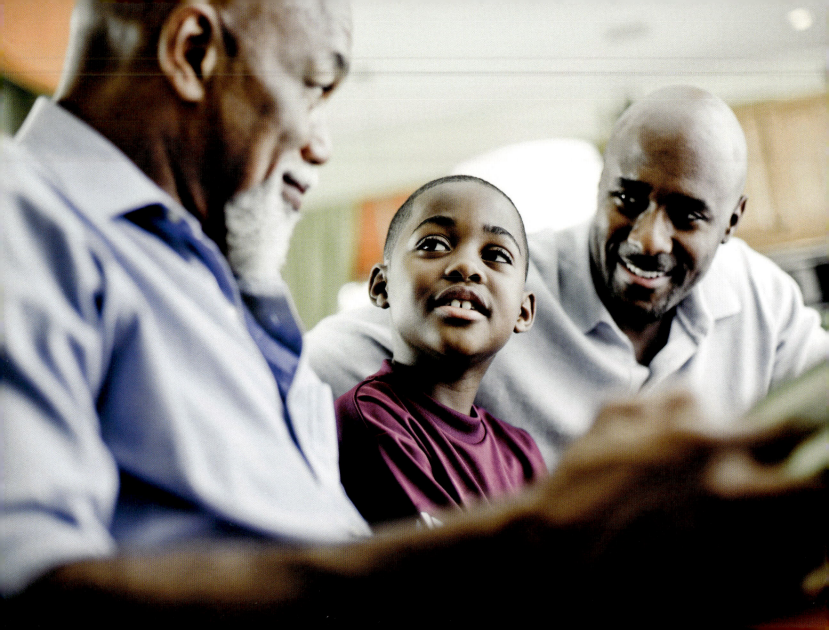

THINK:

1. Does the "lack of time" excuse for not exercising resonate with you? What have you learned that might help you overcome this obstacle?

....

....

....

....

2. Is vigorous-intensity exercise something you are interested in or does it sound like "pain and sweat"? Some people enjoy vigorous-intensity exercise but if that is not you, stay with moderate-intensity—it still delivers great benefits.

....

....

....

DAY 11

LEARN: Read Chapter 4 "Oxygenate": "More is better for staying slim" (page 48).

EXPERIENCE:

1. Your challenge today is simple: achieve a personal best. Determine today to record more steps or VIPs than you have since starting the "Live More: Active" journey. While you are in the process of achieving a personal best, seek out a walking track or course in your area that you can easily access.

THINK:

1. Are you surprised to learn that because we are so inactive nowadays, 30 minutes of moderate-intensity activity a day may not be enough?

....

....

2. Is weight management a concern for you? How much activity do you think you should be aiming for a day?

....

....

EXAMPLES OF HOW TO COUNT VIPs USING THE "EXERCISE METHOD"

Heather made an effort to get out of her seat semi-regularly during the day (5 VIPs). She went for a 40-minute brisk walk in the morning before work at a moderate intensity (4 VIPs), then ducked out for another 10 minutes at lunch time (1 VIP). Heather made the mark—achieving 10 VIPs for the day!

Grace was on her feet for much of the day at work (5 VIPs). She is only starting out on living more active so, for her, a slower walk represents a 3- to 4-out-of-10 in effort (moderate-intensity). Grace parked further from the train station so she had to stroll for 20 minutes in the morning (2 VIPs), then again in the afternoon (2 VIPs). Grace's daily tally equals 9 VIPs. Well done, Grace!

Jason tries to keep moving through the day (5 VIPs). After work, he went swimming for a total of 40 minutes—for the first 20 minutes, he swam at a moderate-intensity (2 VIPs) after which he performed four 5-minute efforts of vigorous-intensity with a rest in between each one (4 VIPs). Jason scores 11 VIPs for the day. Way to go, Jason!

DAY 12

LEARN: Read Chapter 5, "Excuses, excuses!": Excuses 1 to 5 (pages 51-57).

EXPERIENCE:

1. While lack of time is often cited as an excuse for not exercising, I have discovered that exercise can save you time. Today, I would like you to test it out and you have two challenges to choose from:

> *Option 1:* Take a problem you have been struggling with that has consumed much of your time recently or some assignment that will consume much of your time in the future. Give it your full attention while you exercise. Ideally, go for a long walk or jog outside in a "green" space.
>
> *Option 2:* Organize a walk-while-we-talk meeting with someone to discuss an issue that calls for creativity and clear thinking. Dedicate 30 minutes to the task. Get out into a natural environment if you can.

2. Record how many VIPs you achieved for the day in the activity log on page 186.

THINK:

1. Is lack of time an excuse for not exercising that resonates with you? What have you learned that might help you overcome this obstacle?

....

....

....

2. Have you heard stories about the dangers of exercise? From what you have learned, do they seem less founded?

....

....

....

3. Did you discover during today's challenge that you were able to think clearly and creatively on the move? If so, how could you use regular exercise to save you time in the future?

....

....

....

DAY 13

LEARN: Read Chapter 5 "Excuses, excuses!": Excuses 6 to 10 (pages 57-63).

EXPERIENCE:

1. Remember when you were a kid and you "played"? By definition, "play" refers to activities that we do for the sheer enjoyment of it—we don't need any other reward, because it is fun in and of itself. In the animal kingdom, play is considered a sign of intelligence—monkeys play, dolphins play, amoebas don't. What I find fascinating is that children are the masters of play but adults seem to lose the ability. What does that say about us "grown ups"? I want you to rediscover active play.

Your challenge today is to engage in some kind of active play—just for fun. Even if it is only for 10 minutes, build it into your activity time today. If you need help with active play, learn from the play-masters: children. You will find them most welcoming and their enthusiasm is infectious

2. Record how many VIPs you achieved for the day in the activity log on page 186.

THINK:

1. Are there still some things about exercise and being active that you are unclear about? Write them down and be sure to search for the answers if they haven't been answered by the end of this "Live More: Active" journey. Identifying the right questions to ask is the first step toward having them answered!

....

....

....

2. Is exercise becoming less boring for you? What are some things you can do to make it more interesting?

....

....

....

3. How did your play date go?

....

....

....

DAY 14

REST

REST DAY!

The last excuse we looked at yesterday related to feeling embarrassed about exercising. You are now two weeks into the "Live More: Active" challenge and I just want to say that you have nothing to be embarrassed about and everything to be proud of! I celebrate your achievement. Well done!

Everyone is on a journey in terms of their health and fitness, even elite athletes. The fact that you have joined the journey makes you an equal. It is the direction you face—not the position you hold—that is important.

Reward yourself with a rest day. Of course, you can still record how many VIPs you achieve today in the activity log on page 186 if you choose.

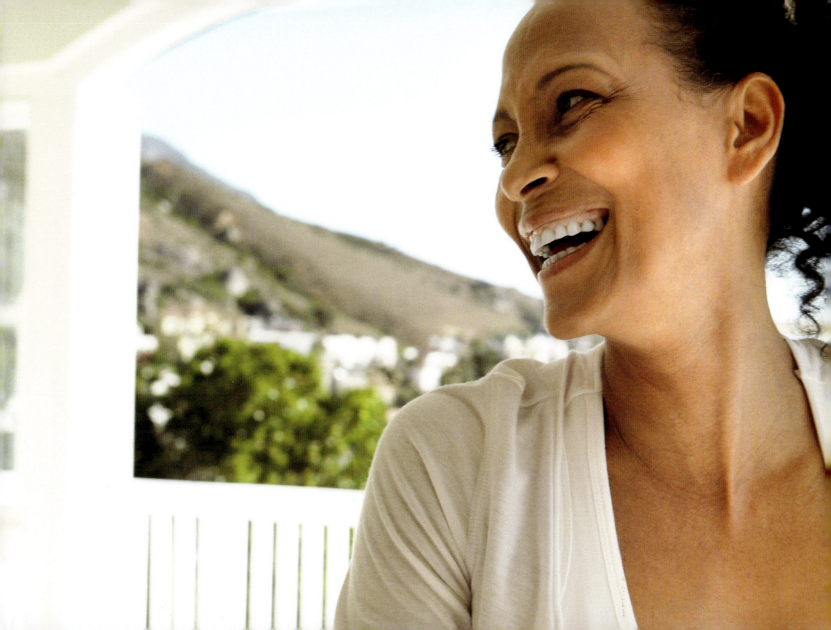

DAY 15

LEARN: Read Chapter 6 "Strengthen and Stretch" (pages 64-90).

EXPERIENCE:

1. Your challenge today involves testing out the resistance exercises you have learned. Hopefully, you are now convinced that resistance exercises are an essential part of your activity routine.

Being mindful to start slowly and careful not to over-extend yourself, select one exercise that is appropriate for you from each of the four "Muscle Action" categories shown in Section 1 (pages 74-90). After a warm-up, which might include 10 minutes of moderate-intensity aerobic activity like a brisk walk or jog, perform one "set" of each of the four exercises.

Remember, you are aiming to select a level of difficulty that you can perform about 12 repetitions. Take breaks of 30-60 seconds between each exercise. Once you have performed all four exercises, repeat the process once more through, performing the exercises in the same order.

Here is how you can score VIPs using resistance exercises: For every four sets of 12 quality repetitions performed—it is OK if you do a few more or less repetitions—you get 1 VIP.

4 sets of approximately 12 quality repetitions = 1 VIP

The routine you did today, which involved a total of eight sets (two sets of each of the four exercises you selected), earned you 2 VIPs. If you did a 10-minute warm up involving moderate-intensity physical activity, you actually scored 3 VIPs!

Note: If you are using the "Steps method" to achieve your daily VIPs, you can still incorporate resistance exercises. For example, you could combine your 2 VIPs from the resistance exercises performed in today's challenge with 8000 steps (or 8 VIPs) to achieve 10 VIPs for the day.

2. Record how many VIPs you achieved today in the activity log on page 187. Note that you are free to perform other moderate-intensity or vigorous-intensity physical activities on days you do resistance exercises to score more VIPs.

THINK:

1. What are some of the benefits of resistance exercises that are personally relevant to you? Are you convinced it is important that you perform them?

....

....

....

2. How did you go with the simple resistance exercises routine you performed today? Does it feel like something you need to do more often?

....

....

....

Live More **ACTIVE** | 165

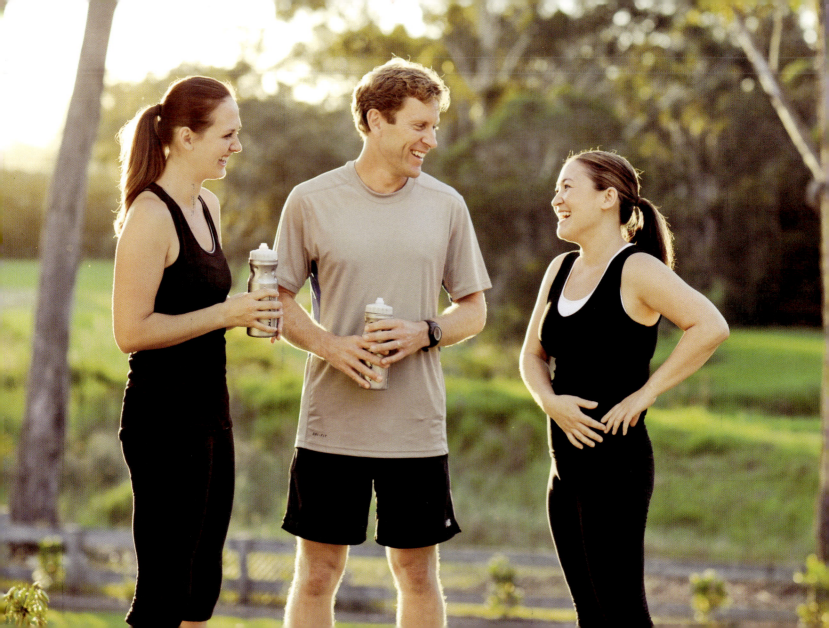

DAY 16

LEARN: Read Chapter 6 "Strengthen and Stretch": "Stretch it out" (pages 91-94).

EXPERIENCE:

1. Take some time today to perform all the stretching exercises for the upper body shown on page 92. For each exercise, hold the stretch for about 20 seconds, rest for 20 seconds, then repeat until you have completed the stretch three times. Then move on to the next stretch.

The bad news is you don't earn any VIPs for the stretching exercises—but the good news is that they are great for you and will make you feel good!

2. Record how many VIPs you achieved today in the activity log on page 187.

THINK:

1. What benefits of stretching are important for you?

....

....

2. How did you feel after stretching? Did you notice that you gained more mobility in the joints as you stretched them? Did you feel more flexible after completing the stretches?

....

....

DAY 17

LEARN: Read Chapter 7 "Moving to success": To "Making your *inside* world work for you" (pages 96-99).

EXPERIENCE: Today you have a physical challenge and a non-physical challenge:

1. First for the physical challenge: Repeat the same four resistance exercises you performed two days ago in the same order, but this time add an extra lap so you perform each exercise three times. In total, you will therefore complete 12 sets, which will earn you 3 VIPs. Remember:

> **4 sets of approximately 12 quality repetitions = 1 VIP**

As you progress and begin to regularly include resistance exercises in your activity program, don't always perform the same exercises. Selecting different exercises from the four "Muscle Action" categories challenges your body in new ways, which causes it to respond positively. Plus, it makes your activity time more interesting as it adds variety.

2. Now for the non-physical challenge: Your reading today asked if you have a knowledge gap. Since beginning this "Live More: Active" challenge, there are bound to be gaps that have already been filled. Write down three things you have learned that have interested and/or helped you:

....

....

....

Your challenge is to share them—with someone else or a group of people. You don't have to make a big deal out of it but just try to work them into a conversation. Hopefully, you have been sharing what you have been learning anyway, but today I am making it part of your challenge!

3. Record how many VIPs you achieved today in the activity log on page 187.

THINK:

1. As you reflected on what you have learned, did it occur to you that you are becoming quite informed about more active living? What information did you share today and with whom?

....

....

....

2. Did you feel better today when performing the resistance exercises than you did two days ago? It is amazing how quickly your strength will improve as you perform resistance exercises more regularly. What did you notice?

....

....

....

DAY 18

LEARN: Read Chapter 7 "Moving to success": "Are you task-orientated?" to "Are you an introvert or extrovert?" (pages 101–103).

EXPERIENCE: We are getting close to the end of the 21-day "Live More: Active" challenge, but what are you going to do after? A really good way to maintain momentum is to have a goal to work toward.

As explained on page 101, the "SMART goals" approach is a good strategy for setting goals. Take the time to create your own SMART goals in the table provided. As you do, here are a couple of other tips:

› Think outside the square. Is there some physical pursuit you have never entertained the idea of doing? Enter a fun run/walk. Try a triathlon. Why not?

› No goal is too small. It is a good idea to have grand long-term goals, but smaller short-term goals can act as stepping-stones along the way.

› Don't be afraid of failure. The only failure is not trying. Everyone fails at times, and these failed attempts can teach us more than our successes. Try again.

› Take your goals seriously. Don't over-commit and don't under-deliver. This will grow your self-belief and personal integrity.

› Reward yourself when you achieve your goals—it reinforces the pleasure associated with doing what you are doing!

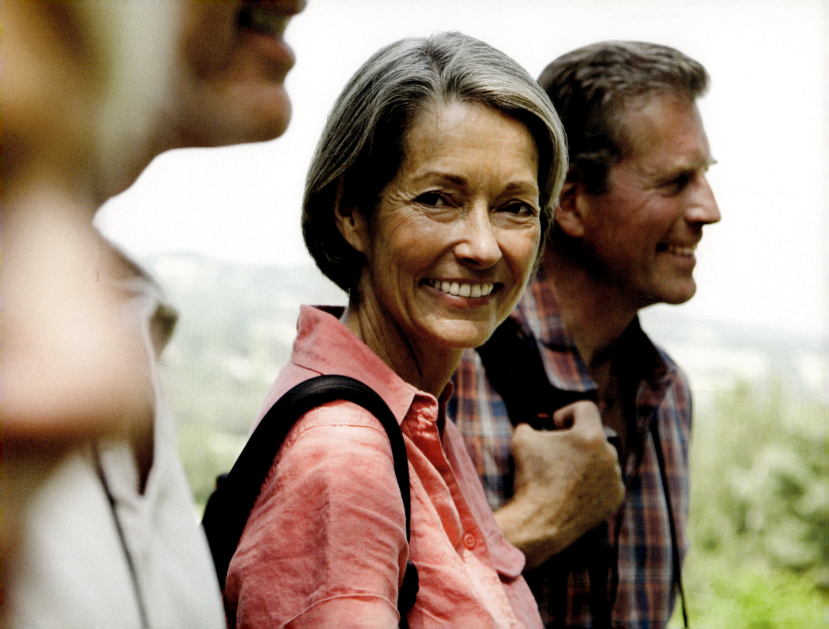

SMART Goals and Action Plan

S — SPECIFIC
What are you going to achieve? What are the steps? This is where your Action Plan comes in handy!

M — MEASURABLE
How will you know that you have achieved your goal? How will others know?

A — ACHIEVABLE
What is needed to achieve this goal? Do you need anyone to help you achieve this goal?

R — RELEVANT
How does your goal relate to your health and wellbeing? What is the reason you would like to achieve this goal?

T — TIMELY
When do you plan to implement and reach your goal?

› Finally, it is a good idea to write the goal as if it is already a reality. Instead of writing "I would like to . . ." say "I am/I can. . . ." We have provided an example below.

[Define when you want to have achieved your goal.]

[The evidence: How you will know that your goal has been reached; your measures?]

TODAY'S DATE	MY GOAL	WHEN?	RESULT
September 28	My fitness level has improved...	By the end of next month . . .	As evidenced by the fact that I can go for a 15 minute jog without stopping.

Action Plan: Steps to achieve your goal

ACTION STEPS Consider specific strategies/methods	HOW WILL I DO THIS? Who is involved/helping you; how often will you do it?	WHEN WILL I DO THIS? When will you do the things?	WHAT DO I NEED TO DO THIS? Equipment, schedule free time, certain ingredients, skills, knowledge, etc.	HOW WILL I KNOW I HAVE DONE IT?
Go for a run (walk when necessary)	For 20 minutes with Katie	At lunch time at least 3 days during the work week	Take sport clothes and shoes to work, pack towel, shower gel, clean socks. Block out time and set automatic calendar reminders. Remind Katie to do the same. Take watch along on runs.	Circle days in calendar that I went for a run and note down the time I spent running. Count the days or weeks it took to reach my 15-minute running goal.

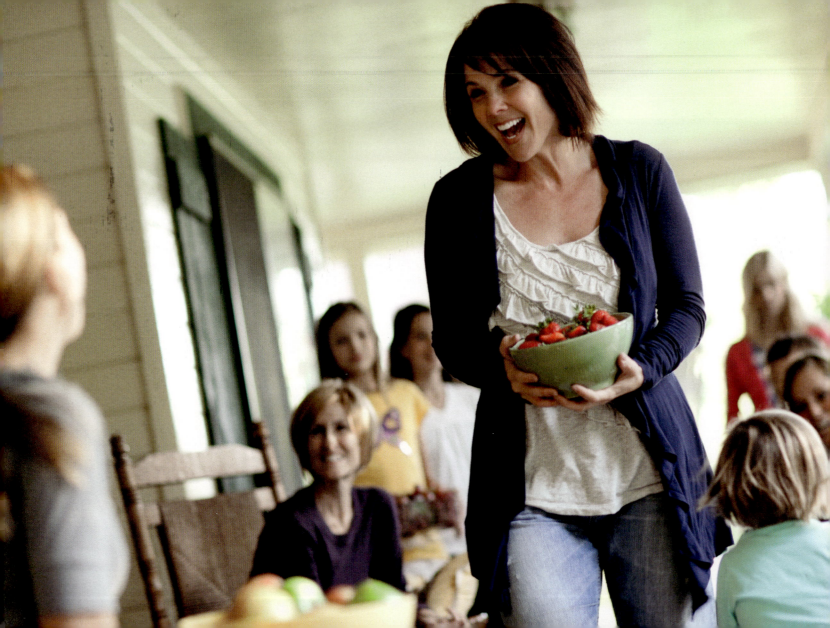

THINK:

1. What times in your life can you remember setting a goal and achieving it (it doesn't have to be in relation to physical activity)? How did that make you feel?

....

....

....

2. If an introvert is energized by their own company, while an extrovert is recharged by the company of others, which are you? How could you use this realization to make your exercise time more enjoyable?

....

....

....

3. You now have a goal(s) to work toward. How confident are you that you can achieve them? You are capable of more than you realize!

....

....

....

DAY 19

LEARN: Read Chapter 7 "Moving to success": "Do you enjoy structure or variety?" and "Are other lifestyle practices making it harder for you to be physically active?" (pages 104-105).

EXPERIENCE: As we have learned, being physically active is one of the best things you can do for your health and wellbeing. However, other lifestyle practices also make a huge difference to your level of vitality. Your eating pattern is one vital factor.

Your challenge today is to "fiber up." The simplest strategy for improving your diet is to prioritize foods that are naturally high in fiber and minimize those that aren't. High-fiber foods are high in all the "good stuff," including vitamins, minerals and antioxidants. They are also low in—or free from—the "bad stuff," including saturated fats and cholesterol.

So what does a high-fiber diet look like? For starters, fiber is only found in plant foods. There is no fiber in any animal products, including meat, eggs, dairy and fish. Also, when foods are processed, much of the fiber is robbed from them. In summary, a high-fiber diet is rich in plant foods, such as fruits, grains, vegetables and legumes, that are minimally processed—the ideal being "foods-as-grown."

Today, I want you to eat more! That is, eat more of the high-fiber foods by putting an unprocessed plant slant to your diet. Here are some simple ideas for achieving it:

> *Have a hearty breakfast with wholegrain cereals and fruit.*
> *Opt for wholegrain breads and brown rice, rather than the white varieties.*
> *Snack on natural fruit and vegetables, such as apples or carrot sticks.*

If you are up for a real challenge, test out this pattern of eating for a few days. You will be amazed at how much better you will feel.

Note: A high-fiber diet can get you on the move in more ways than one—constipation becomes a thing of the past! So be sure to keep drinking your eight glasses of water a day.

THINK:

1. What other lifestyle changes could you benefit from?

....

....

....

....

2. How did you go with the "fiber up" challenge? Did you notice things start to move? If not, wait until tomorrow! Do you feel better for it?

....

....

....

....

DAY 20

LEARN: Read Chapter 7 "Moving to success": "Making your outside world work for you" to "You're on the journey" (pages 106-110).

EXPERIENCE: Today you have two challenges:

1. Include resistance exercises in your activity time, but this time in a slightly different way. First, select an exercise from each of the four "Muscle Action" categories (ideally one you haven't completed as yet). Perform each of the four exercises either two or three times but instead of just resting between the sets, add in an activity that "oxygenates," for example, a brisk walk, jog, skip or stationary cycle for two minutes.
The pattern would be:

- Oxygenate for 2 minutes
- Muscle Action category 1 exercise
- Oxygenate for 2 minutes
- Muscle Action category 2 exercise
- Oxygenate for 2 minutes
- Muscle Action category 3 exercise
- Oxygenate for 2 minutes
- Muscle Action category 4 exercise

Repeat two or three times.

This style of exercise is called "circuit training" and provides a complete workout. Because it is quite energetic, it can typically be considered "vigorous-intensity" activity, which makes it a time-efficient way of achieving VIPs, earning 1 VIP for every five minutes of the circuit training described above.

2. Are there any physical activities you have always thought would be fun to try but you have never got around to? Are there physical activities you enjoyed as a "younger person" but have not engaged in for many years? Your challenge today is to insert some active fun into your life. You don't have to perform the activity today but you must take action toward it. Here are some ideas:

> ❯ *Inquire about a local hiking group.*
>
> ❯ *Try a round of golf (and don't hire a buggy!).*
>
> ❯ *Enter a fun run/walk or triathlon.*
>
> ❯ *Join a local sporting club (check out the "Masters" sports and games—you don't have to be that old).*

You are never too old for fun and there are bound to be opportunities in your area that you haven't considered. Discover them.

THINK:

1. Are you surprised to learn how powerful social influences can be on your health and wellbeing? Who do you know that models the kind of health behaviors you would like to adopt?

....

....

....

2. Can you identify examples in your local community that illustrate how a change in the physical environment can influence people's activity levels—for good or bad?

....

....

....

3. Can you identify any changes that could be made in your local area to empower others to live more active?

....

....

....

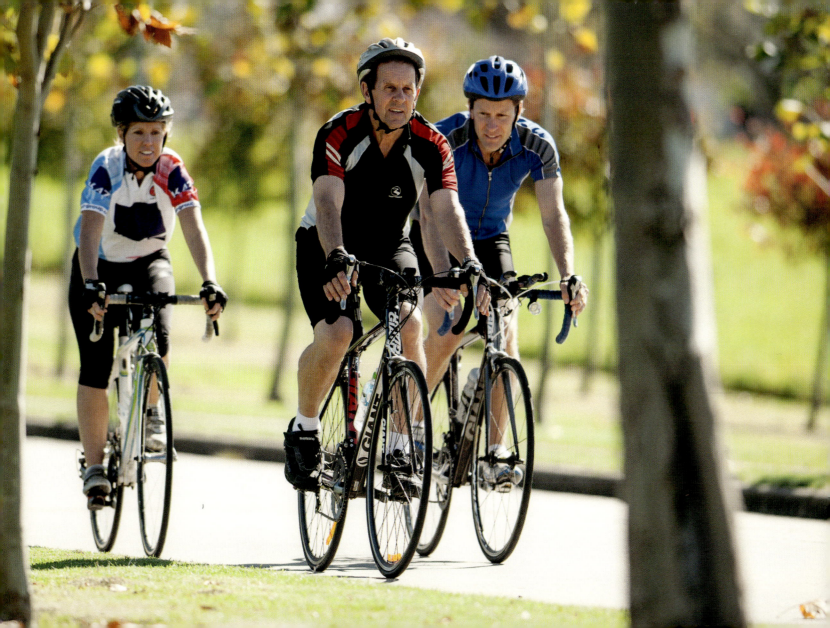

DAY 21

LEARN: Read Chapter 8 "The power of belief" (pages 112-120).

EXPERIENCE: Respond to the challenge on page 118 and become an agent of change.

List three changes you can make to your environment to help support your intention to live more active. Your job is to find the subtle—and not-so-subtle—ways the world about you currently enables old sedentary habits, then redesign it to support your goals to become active. If the changes you make help others become more active too, then great!

1. ....

2. ....

3. ....

THINK:

1. Do you agree that beliefs drive behavior?

....

....

....

2. Honestly, do you believe you *need* to be active, you *can* be active, and you *deserve* to be active and enjoy the associated benefits?

....

....

....

3. Reflecting back on your journey over the past 21 days, what three things have gone well? How does it make you feel when you think about these positive experiences and/or achievements?

....

....

....

A FINAL WORD

Congratulations on getting to Day 21 and making it through the "Live More: Active" challenge. You should be proud! The intent of this 21-day activation was to kick-start you to live more active—and you are off to a great start.

But, of course, this is just the beginning of the journey. You are equipped with all the information and strategies you need to activate your life for good, so keep moving forward. Aim to achieve 10 VIPs a day (or 50 to 70 VIPs a week) as you Sit less, Oxygenate, and Strengthen and stretch. Be sure to include all elements!

As Pythagoras asserted, "Keep choosing what is best; habit will soon render it agreeable and easy." Living more active is an integral part of living your best life.

Live more.

Darren Morton

1,000 steps = 1 VIP

5 VIPs for not sitting too much

10 minutes = 1 VIP

5 minutes = 1 VIP

4 sets = 1 VIP

DAY	STEPS METHOD		EXERCISE METHOD							
	STEP COUNT	TOTAL VIPs	BONUS VIPs	MODERATE INTENSITY MINUTES	VIPs	VIGOROUS INTENSITY MINUTES	VIPs	RESISTANCE EXERCISE SETS	VIPs	TOTAL VIPs
1			5							
2			5							
3			5							
4			5							
5			5							
6			5							
7			5							

WEEKLY TOTAL VIPs = _____

Total your daily VIPs achieved using the Exercise Method by:
5 Bonus VIPs + Moderate VIPs + Vigorous VIPs + Resistance VIPs

Live More ACTIVE

DAY	STEPS METHOD		EXERCISE METHOD						
	STEP COUNT	TOTAL VIPs	BONUS VIPs	MODERATE INTENSITY		VIGOROUS INTENSITY		RESISTANCE EXERCISE		TOTAL VIPs
				MINUTES	VIPs	MINUTES	VIPs	SETS	VIPs	
8			5							
9			5							
10			5							
11			5							
12			5							
13			5							
14			5							

WEEKLY TOTAL VIPs = _____

DAY	STEPS METHOD		EXERCISE METHOD							
	STEP COUNT	TOTAL VIPs	BONUS VIPs	MODERATE INTENSITY MINUTES	VIPs	VIGOROUS INTENSITY MINUTES	VIPs	RESISTANCE EXERCISE SETS	VIPs	TOTAL VIPs
15			5							
16			5							
17			5							
18			5							
19			5							
20			5							
21			5							

WEEKLY TOTAL VIPs = _____

Live More **ACTIVE**

Prevent, arrest and even reverse chronic disease

COMPLETE HEALTH IMPROVEMENT PROGRAM

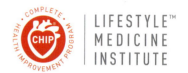

Most people today live with chronic health problems and die too soon from chronic diseases and their complications. I am talking about heart disease, stroke, cancers, and type 2 diabetes. Yet we know that these are lifestyle related. In fact, up to 90 per cent of heart disease and type 2 diabetes is preventable. But the exciting thing is that there is hope, not just for prevention or management of disease, but in some instances, chronic diseases can even be reversed.

I am part of the team from the not-for-profit Lifestyle Medicine Institute responsible for the development and distribution of the global lifestyle intervention known as CHIP—the Complete Health Improvement Program.

CHIP is a group-based lifestyle program designed to prevent, arrest and even reverse many of the ill-health conditions that plague us today. It provides the education, motivation, support and friendship necessary to turn your life around. And what is so unique about CHIP is that it adopts a whole-of-health approach by addressing all aspects of wellbeing, including nutrition, physical activity, substance use, stress, self-worth, and even happiness—after all, what's the point of being healthy if you're miserable? CHIP gives people all the pieces of the puzzle required to truly flourish and indeed CHIP is giving people their life back around the globe.

As a presenter of CHIP and also one who is actively involved in researching its effectiveness, I can tell you that CHIP achieves priceless benefits and proven results. We have published many studies demonstrating the effectiveness of CHIP in prestigious peer-reviewed, academic journals such as the *American Journal of Cardiology*. So I can tell you with confidence that CHIP works.

If you would like to learn more about CHIP, get on to the CHIP website—<www.CHIPhealth.com>—and join me on this exciting journey to better living and better health.

Darren Morton

Darren Morton, PhD
Lifestyle Research Centre
Avondale College of Higher Education

www.chiphealth.com

PROVEN RESULTS™
Priceless benefits